ABOUT THE EDITORS

Susan Bird BA(Nurs) RGN CCNS CertEd (FE) FRSH

Susan Bird is a graduate nurse and depute head of department in James Watt College, Greenock. She was formerly Regional Coordinator for Open Learning, Strathclyde Regional Council and has taught in Further Education for several years. She is also a verifier in caring for SCOTVEC (Scottish Vocational Educational Council) and previously worked with SCOTVEC as National Development Officer for the Support Worker (Nursing) Programme and as a Project Officer for the National Health Service Training Authority (NHSTA) Health Care Support Worker Project and the Residential, Domiciliary and Day Care Project (RDDC).

David Rennie DYCS DSW CQSW

David Rennie is professionally qualified in social work and community work and has had extensive experience in social work as a practitioner, manager and trainer. He is a Mental Health Officer (Approved Social Worker) and helped design Strathclyde Regional Council's mental health training programme. He was seconded to the Care Sector Consortium to research and develop the new National Standards for social care workers and worked as a Development Officer with SCOTVEC. He is presently Inspector with the Inspection Unit of Strathclyde Regional Council Social Work Department, which has responsibility for inspecting residential social work establishments across the statutory, voluntary and private sectors.

ABOUT THE AUTHORS

Margaret Miller RGN SCM CertEd(FE)

Margaret Miller has worked for many years teaching health subjects to students in further education. She is currently employed by Jordanhill College in the Scottish School of Further Education. She is also a member of the Institute of Transactional Analysis and a representative for TA in Education in Scotland.

Janet Campbell BA(SocSci) RGN SCM HV Cert FWT CertEd(FE)

Janet Campbell teaches general nurse students at Argyll and Clyde College of Nursing and Midwifery and is a guest lecturer in communications at Paisley College. She gratefully acknowledges the assistance of Argyll and Clyde Health Board, and Mrs Anthony, CANO, in allowing her time to work on her contribution to this book.

Joan Garrigan BSc(Hons) RGN CMB HV Cert(HealthEd)

Joan Garrigan is a Health Visitor in Glasgow and is currently completing a BSc (Hons) in Health Studies at Queen's College, Glasgow.

ABOUT THE OPEN LEARNING ADVISOR

Glennis Johnson BSc

Glennis Johnson is an educationalist with wide experience in Further Education and in the preparation and development of Open Learning materials. She was previously Programme Manager, then advisor and editor, to the Continuing Nurse Education Programme series of Open Learning Material produced by Barnet College.

ABOUT TERMINOLOGY

Throughout the text the recipients of all types of care are referred to as 'clients' and those involved in providing the care as 'care workers'. For simplicity, clients are always referred to as 'he' and care workers as 'she'.

HUMAN DEVELOPMENT

Margaret Miller
RGN SCM CertEd(FE)

Janet Campbell
BA RGN SCM HV Cert FWT CertEd(FE)

Joan Garrigan
BSc(Hons) RGN CMB HV Cert(HealthEd)

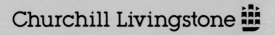

Churchill Livingstone

EDINBURGH LONDON MADRID MELBOURNE NEW YORK AND TOKYO 1992

CHURCHILL LIVINGSTONE
Medical Division of Longman Group UK Limited

Distributed in the United States of America by Churchill
Livingstone Inc., 1560 Broadway, New York, NY 10036, and by
associated companies, branches and representatives
throughout the world.

First published 1992

ISBN 0-443-04531-3

British Library Cataloguing In Publication Data
A catalogue record for this book is available from the British
Library.

Library of Congress Cataloging in Publication Data
A catalog record for this book is available from the Library of
Congress.

For Churchill Livingstone

Publisher: Mary Law
Project Manager: Ellen Green
Editor: Valerie Bain
Production Controller: Nancy Henry
Design: Design Resources Unit
Sales Promotion Executive: Hilary Brown

Produced by Longman Singapore Publishers Pte Ltd
Printed in Singapore

Contents

Introduction   *1*

1   *What is human development?* *2*

2   *Areas of development* *6*

3   *Conception to birth*   *10*

4   *Infancy*   *18*

5   *Childhood years*   *22*

6   *Adolescence*   *27*

7   *Adulthood*   *33*

8   *The middle years*   *37*

9   *The older adult*   *40*

Answers   *47*

To the reader

Here are some questions which may occur to you before you start to read this book

Who is this book for?
Anyone involved in caring. It has been designed with you – the reader – in mind. We've tried to make it look and feel friendly and attractive.

Do I need to enrol in a course to use this book?
Certainly not, although you may find that it is used by many Caring courses. The books in the **Skills for Caring** series are for anyone involved in caring. You can use it on your own, at your workplace as part of an assessment programme if you're in employment, or as part of a more formal training programme at a college or other institution.

Where can I read this book?
Anywhere you like. You can read it in 'snatches', if this is more convenient for you, or you can interrupt your reading to do some of the exercises. It may help you to write on it, if it's your own copy. As you will see, the book has been designed to be used in a very flexible way.

Are there any special features that I should be aware of before starting to read this book?
You'll find it a great help to know the following:

Definitions:
Sometimes a key word might be unfamiliar to some readers, or we might want to be sure that the **precise** meaning is clear. We've tried to pick out such words and give their meaning at the place where the word is first mentioned. The word and its definition have been set off in a box.

Examples:
There's no substitute for a good example to make a point or convey a message. We've included as many examples as possible and have set these off from the main text with boxes, so that you can skip them if you like, or locate them again if you found them particularly helpful.

Exercises:
These have been set off from the text in a different colour. The exercises can extend your knowledge considerably and reinforce what you've read in the main text. You can do the exercises on your own, with a group, or under the direction of a tutor. Or you can choose **not** to do them at all, or to do them later, after you've read and absorbed the text. The choice is yours. Remember: this is **your** book – enjoy it!

Introduction

◾ *Caring is about people, whatever their age, race, sex, marital status, social class or shoe size! It involves individuals – those who do the caring and those in need of care.*

Human development continues all through our lives and every individual is somewhere on the track, either on the starting blocks or heading towards the finishing line. As a carer, you may become involved with people at any stage of this process and in many situations in the home, a hospital or the community. You may work as a health service employee, on a voluntary basis or in another capacity but, irrespective of who or where they are, those in need of care are individuals.

This book will help you gain knowledge and understanding of the human development process so that you can become more aware of what influences us as individuals.

It is important to remember, however, that although this book presents a basic, factual account of the human development process, **human development is unique to the individual**. A factual account may, for example, stereotype elderly people as retired, white-haired, wearing glasses and having false teeth, but not all elderly people fit into that picture, especially nowadays. Some older people take on new ventures, roles and occupations when they retire.

In this book we have taken examples from the different stages of the life process and presented the kinds of changes and behaviours you can expect to encounter. However, you may find that *your* experience of people at these stages is slightly different.

Things can go wrong and interfere with the development process. If you are interested in finding out more about any of these topics, you can get information from a library, especially one linked to a health and social studies education or training establishment. A tutor or librarian will help you find suitable books.

We have suggested a few other book resources to help you with your study. If these are not the style of text you enjoy reading there are many other relevant books which will provide an up-to-date view of statistics, diagnoses, signs and symptoms and management of specific problems. These, and other books which you will find useful throughout your study, are listed at the end of the book.

Answers to exercises

Many different kinds of exercise have been used throughout this book. Some are about people you know (Ex. 1) or about you as an individual (Ex. 5) and your opinions (Ex 18). Some ask you to use information from the text (Ex. 6) or to do some further research using other textbooks (Ex. 9).

Where appropriate, we have given guidelines to answers in the text after an exercise. Otherwise, suggested answers can be found in small type at the back of the book.

1

What is human development?

THE MEANING OF 'DEVELOPMENT'

What do we mean by 'development'? You might have used it about everyday things, like the development of a new product or machine, meaning something which is carefully designed to carry out specific functions and which is able to cope with all the demands made on it.

In many ways, that is what the human body is – a machine designed to carry out a series of very difficult tasks. Long before birth the engineering is designed. The process starts at conception, the beginning of a new life, and continues as the human being proceeds through the stages of pre-birth, birth, infancy, childhood, adolescence and adulthood. As well as an increase in body size, which is called growth, progressive changes in body structure, and in the brain, occur as we gain and use knowledge and develop skills. This process is called **development** and it results in an individual person – we are all different.

DEVELOPMENT POTENTIAL

At first, we are very dependent on other adults to supply our needs and are influenced by the environment, or surroundings, in which we live and grow. But, as we grow, we should become less dependent, build on our childhood experiences and take advantage of the opportunities available to us which allow us to achieve full potential. Even those who are in some way disadvantaged mentally or physically can achieve their *individual* maximum development potential with appropriate support from others.

Each normal human being is born with the same basic structures which allow the body to carry out its functions. If, for example, we were to look at a 1000 normal, newborn babies, we would find that all of them perform exactly the same functions. They feed, sleep, soil and cry. The differences between them are in relation to appearance, for example, their weight, skin colour, hair colour and body shape. These are the characteristics that are passed on from parents by what we call **heredity**.

From birth we constantly interact and establish relationships with our fellow human beings. The human infant is more helpless, and matures more slowly, than infants of any other species. As they mature, children behave and develop like those closest to them, for example, their family and friends. These people act as 'role models' and influence our feelings, thoughts and behaviours.

INTERACT: TO HAVE AN EFFECT ON EACH OTHER.

To understand how people interact with their environment we need to know a little about how the nervous and endocrine systems function to coordinate and control our behaviour. As we develop from infancy through adolescence to adulthood, our abilities, attitudes and personalities are moulded together by the situations which we face at different stages of life. This is called our **psychosocial development.**

Babies grow up to achieve different standards of physical performance, that is, **physical development,** and different intellectual levels, that is, **cognitive development**. *You can see this for yourself when you try Exercise 1.*

EXERCISE 1

- Think of three families who share the same village or street with you. Make a list of all the things you know they can do, either during their work or in their leisure time.
- Make a list of the individuals in your own family:
  - What do they look like?
  - What do they do?
  - How do they spend their time?

- Ask them:
  - What were their ambitions as young children?
  - Would they say that they had fulfilled any of their ambitions?

- If they answer 'No':
  - Why did they not achieve some of the things they had hoped for in the past?
  - Are there things in life that they feel they can still achieve?

The results of Exercise 1 will show enormous variations between individuals. Some people may have fulfilled their ambitions, others will still be striving to achieve them and some may have abandoned the struggle to achieve their goals (like playing football for their country!).

So, although at birth we all seem to have the same machinery and tools to carry out the same body processes and functions, the effects of 'nature' and 'nurture' determine whether or not we achieve our life goals. **Nature**, or heredity, is passed on to us by our parents; **nurture** is the effect of the environment in which we are reared.

As we gain knowledge and skills, and develop our own feelings and attitudes, we are able to make conscious decisions about our own lives. Provided we are healthy and normal, we can set goals and seek out opportunities. Some of these may seem unrealistic because we do not have the resources, either from nature or nurture. However, many people with determination and guidance have achieved goals which might, at one stage, have seemed unrealistic. This is what **development potential** means – the power to develop as far as our abilities allow.

INFLUENCES ON DEVELOPMENT

There are three main factors which influence development at all stages:

- Heredity
- Environment
- Health

HEREDITY

Heredity is a major influence on human development.

> HEREDITY: THE ABILITY OF LIVING THINGS TO PASS ON THEIR OWN CHARACTERISTIC FEATURES FROM PARENT TO CHILD IN THE CELLS OF THE BODY.

Our parents received their characteristics from *their* parents – heredity goes back through generations of families. As partnerships are formed between quite different families, each with their own family trees, the possible variations are endless. *See Exercise 2.*

EXERCISE 2

- Select four people, not from the same family, whom you know very well, and make a list of all the differences between each of them.
- Now take a look at the members of your own family. Are there any features which you have in common with them?

The characteristics we inherit are carried in our **genes** and in Chapter 3, which is about reproduction, we shall look more closely at the influence of genes on human development.

ENVIRONMENT

The environment is anything inside or outside the body to which the body responds. Inside the body, for example, there are temperature changes, chemical changes and the effect of drugs, alcohol or nicotine. Outside the body is the physical environment, things of a material nature that surround us wherever we are at a particular time. *You can think about this further in Exercise 3.*

● ●

EXERCISE 3

- What kind of environment are you in as you read this book? You may be on a plane or bus, in a classroom, in the garden, in your own living room or in the bath.
- Take a look around and consider all the things that might make up the physical environment at present. Don't forget things like heat, light or ventilation.

● ●

There are different types of environment :

- *Socioeconomic environment* **includes the structure of the family unit, the number at work, those unemployed, the number of children, and the interrelationships existing at home, in school or at work.**
- *The intellectual environment* **includes things around us that stimulate us to think, communicate, read, watch, explore and experiment.**
- *The psychosocial environment* **is the effect relationships, feelings and emotions have on our personalities, for example, joy and pleasure from affection, anxiety surrounding going to college or the confidence which comes from doing a good job.**

A human being has the ability to perceive, or make sense of, the environment and no two individuals have exactly the same perceptions of a shared environment. This applies even to identical twins.

Imagine, for example, two people going to a swimming pool. One can swim but the other cannot. The swimmer will experience pleasure and lots of activity; the non-swimmer will feel scared and cling to the side of the pool. You will be able to think of many other situations in the home, in school, at work or at play where you and others react differently to the environment you are all sharing.

HEALTH

Even before conception the health of both parents has a significant influence on whether or not the process of development starts at all. (The process of fertilisation is discussed in Chapter 3.) During pregnancy it is vital that the mother maintains good health; the developing embryo, later the **fetus**, is entirely dependent on the mother for food and for getting rid of waste products. It is therefore particularly vulnerable to any substance the mother introduces into her body which has harmful effects. Once the child is born it is totally dependent on the adult to provide the appropriate food, exercise, rest, sleep, clothing and cleanliness essential to good health. As the process of development continues into adolescence and adulthood, having a healthy lifestyle could have a major influence on ageing.

How we achieve a healthy lifestyle is closely related to the way in which our different needs are met. In the 1950s, a psychologist called Abraham Maslow proposed a theory which is still widely accepted. It suggests that human behaviour and development depend on certain needs being met. These needs can be arranged in a graded order (or hierarchy) from the lowest to the highest level. If needs at the lowest level are not met, then the individual cannot easily move further up the order. (See Figure 1.)

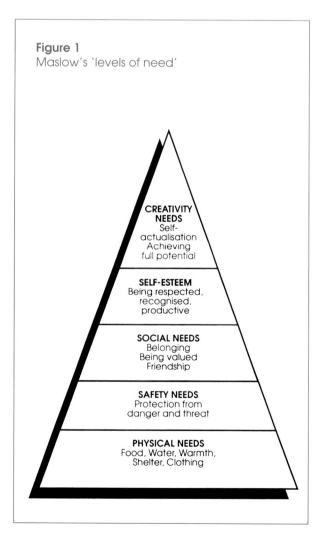

Figure 1
Maslow's 'levels of need'

CREATIVITY NEEDS
Self-actualisation
Achieving full potential

SELF-ESTEEM
Being respected, recognised, productive

SOCIAL NEEDS
Belonging
Being valued
Friendship

SAFETY NEEDS
Protection from danger and threat

PHYSICAL NEEDS
Food, Water, Warmth, Shelter, Clothing

Not all psychologists agree with Maslow's theory, and you may know people who have achieved a higher level of need without meeting the more basic ones. For example, you may feel that although you have very little money to give you security, you have still pursued many interests which have given you pleasure and a sense of achievement (self-actualisation). However, have you ever said to yourself something like 'If only I could afford it I would like to take a university degree or set up my own business.' Some people need to have financial security and will do without food, clothing and warmth to have money in store. They have reversed the process defined by Maslow and run the risk of diseases and illness caused by lack of proper food and body warmth.

SUMMARY EXERCISE

Which of the following would you consider as part of the
- physical environment (A)
- socioeconomic environment (B)
- intellectual environment (C)
- psychosocial environment (D)?

Put A, B, C, or D against the appropriate statements:

- Daily Newspapers being delivered to your home ( )
- A child with lots of books to read ( )
- A home with central heating ( )
- A family where both parents are in employment ( )
- A comfortable bed in which to sleep ( )
- Space in which to take exercise ( )
- Lots of friends to go out with ( )
- A town with high unemployment ( )

(Answers on page 47)

2

Areas of development

■ This chapter explores the different areas of development. Information about human development is usually classified as physical, intellectual, emotional and social development, or as physical and psychosocial development.

PHYSICAL DEVELOPMENT

This area deals with the development of the body. It includes all the structures of the body, their relationship to each other, how they develop and mature, and how they are influenced by factors both within and outside the body.

BASIC STRUCTURES OF THE BODY

The unit of life is called the **cell.** All living creatures start off as a tiny single cell. Our bodies are made up of millions and millions of cells. Groups of cells, like nerve cells or skin cells, are programmed to carry out specific functions, and when they work together in this way we call the specialised group a **tissue.** Bone, muscle, skin and nerves are examples of tissues. Different tissues also form partnerships with each other to carry out more complex body processes and groups of tissues come together to form larger structures called **organs**. Examples of organs are the heart, lungs and kidneys.

The body carries out many specific functions and often we are not aware of these happening, for example, digestion of food, accumulation of waste products for excretion, exchange of gases and function of glands. All these procedures require a highly organised mechanism. To achieve this organs are grouped together into **systems.** For example:

- **nervous system (brain and nerves)**
- **respiratory system (nose, air passages, lungs)**
- **reproductive system (ovaries, uterus and supporting structures in the female).**

PHYSICAL GROWTH

Development begins in the reproductive system, the organs which allow human life to continue.

Physical growth and development are time-related. The experiences from which we learn and grow happen to us at different times, which is why development is referred to as a **process** – it takes time. Also the developing human being does not make very obvious jumps from one stage to the next; the process of physical development is very gradual. Although we know that there are times when growth is more rapid than others we do not actually *see* someone grow taller overnight!

Growth is an increase in size. It involves the areas of height, weight and girth. The pattern varies because these areas may increase in size independently of each other and so the ratio can vary.

> RATIO: THE RELATIONSHIP BETWEEN TWO AMOUNTS, WORKED OUT BY THE NUMBER OF TIMES ONE CONTAINS THE OTHER.

Development is a total body process in which all the areas interlink, or overlap, throughout the person's life-span. This allows the body to mature and so the individual is able to use the body more effectively to achieve increasingly difficult tasks. A 4-year-old child might ride a tricycle but a newborn baby could not, and an adult could manipulate a bicycle, or drive a car. To drive a car, an individual has to use many highly developed mental and physical skills.

To find a way of measuring this process we can examine each area individually using **milestones** and then link them together.

For example, if we took 100 1 year olds and investigated how many of them could stand and walk with help, we might find that 60 of them could. This does not mean that the other 40 are abnormal. If we took 100 children at 18 months and examined them we might find that only 1 or 2 were unable to walk with assistance. Again, they may not be abnormal but they are perhaps a little outside the normal pattern. It may be that they have achieved milestones earlier than is usual in other areas of development.

Milestones are therefore *expected* patterns of development achievement that are used only as a guide, not immediately as a means of stating what is normal or abnormal. However, if a child is 6 months to a year outside the normal, then it is important to recognise this so that some investigation can be carried out to find the explanation. Often, when the cause is identified, something can be done to help the child in the area of poor development.

Nowadays, when a child's development is assessed in the early stages, perhaps at a child health clinic, the following broad heading areas provide the framework for the assessment to be carried out (see Figure 2):

- **posture and large motor skills**
- **vision and fine motor skills**
- **hearing and language**
- **social behaviour and play.**

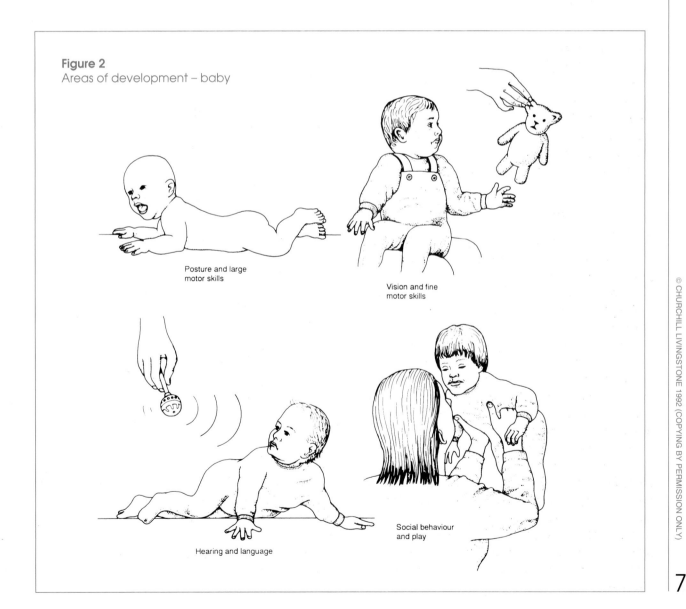

Figure 2
Areas of development – baby

Posture and large
motor skills

Vision and fine
motor skills

Hearing and language

Social behaviour
and play

The same parallels of development are used throughout the child's life and, with modifications, in adulthood as well. For instance, school children may be assessed, perhaps because of a failure to progress, by a multi-disciplinary team comprised of many trained people such as teachers, doctors and psychologists.

See Exercise 4.

● ●

EXERCISE 4

Read the following two case studies then try to work out which experts might be invited to suggest ways of managing the problems involved.

- Janet is a 7 year old in a primary school. She seems a bright, happy individual. When she copies things down in her book she produces very odd images, quite different from anyone else in her class.

- John is at nursery school and his parents expect him to progress to primary school in a few months' time. He seems very interested in all the play activities but everyone finds him difficult to understand. He does not speak clearly and sometimes not at all, making strange noises instead of words. Many of his peers (those children at the same age and stage) have the odd 'accident' in the playroom, but John needs to have several changes of underpants and trousers every day.

(Answers on page 47)

● ●

PSYCHOSOCIAL AND COGNITIVE DEVELOPMENT

PERCEPTION

When we talk of our minds, we normally mean the conscious thoughts, feelings and memories that we are aware of and which guide our actions. Information about our world is registered by our sense organs of sight, sound, smell, taste and touch. This process is known as **perception**; what we perceive is built up in our thought processes into meaningful information so it is totally dependent on our life's experiences.

We acquire our skills and knowledge by learning, remembering and thinking, then we use them to communicate and solve problems. Our behaviour is directed by our motivation and emotions. Our basic motives give us the instinct to survive and direct us towards satisfying our basic needs (see Maslow's hierarchy, page 4). Not only do we have basic needs but we also have social needs of belonging and caring for each other.

Our emotions are the most basic feelings of love, hate, fear, worry, anger, sadness and joy. Emotion triggers our **autonomic nervous system**, that part of our nervous system which is outside our control and which brings about bodily changes, such as rapid heart beat and breathing, dryness of the mouth and throat, increased muscle tension, perspiration, trembling and a 'sinking' feeling in the stomach. This prepares the body for 'fight or flight', whichever is necessary for survival. However, if there is no physical activity to release this pent-up anxiety, it will be experienced as muscle tension. If this happens over a long period then we suffer from too much **stress**.

How are you affected by stress? Try Exercise 5.

● ●

EXERCISE 5

List these stressful life events in the order of importance to you:
- death of a spouse
- divorce
- marital separation
- jail sentence
- death of a close family member
- personal injury or illness
- marriage
- loss of job/redundancy
- marital reconciliation
- retirement
- pregnancy
- new family member
- death of a close friend
- change of job
- child leaving home
- trouble with in-laws
- beginning/ending school
- moving house
- changing schools
- change in sleeping habits
- change in eating habits
- holidays
- Christmas.

If possible, compare your results with someone else. Do you agree with one another?

● ●

When you complete Exercise 5 you will probably discover that, just as emotions affect people in different ways so, too, do life events – we all react differently to, for example, parenthood or job loss.

STAGES OF COGNITIVE DEVELOPMENT

Jean Piaget (1896-1980), a Swiss psychologist, studied the way in which children make sense of their world by dealing actively with objects and people. As children matured from babies to adults, he saw that their intellectual development passed through various stages which he described as 'cognitive development' or 'knowledge building'.

Cognitive development passes through four recognised stages, each stage following on the previous one. These stages are shown in the panel in the left-hand column. Under 2 years of age the baby learns by means of his senses and his own actions. Memory is only beginning to develop and he cannot reason why things happen. Children think differently from adults and should not be regarded as miniature adults.

LEARNING THEORY

There is no such thing as an 'ideal' adult – we are all a result of what we learn throughout life. Learning is the process by which our behaviour is modified, or changed, as a result of our experiences. Our behaviour can be changed by conditioning, that is, our response to a situation depends on our previous experiences. Experiences, including rewards and punishments, change our behaviour, for example, we know not to touch a hot fire because of the consequences – we get burned! Our behaviour can also be changed by observing the behaviour; of others; this is known as 'observed learning'. Not all behaviour is learned; some of our responses are reflex actions, such as blinking and swallowing.

PIAGET'S STAGES OF COGNITIVE DEVELOPMENT

STAGE – **Sensorimotor**
AGE – Birth to 2 years
CHARACTERISATION – Differentiates self from objects.
Recognises self as agent of action and begins to act intentionally, e.g. pulls a string to set a toy in action.
Realises that objects exist even when no longer present to the senses.

STAGE – **Pre-operational**
AGE – 2-7 years approximately
CHARACTERISATION – Learns to use language and to represent objects by images and words, e.g. make-believe play.
Self-centred, unable to see other's point of view.

STAGE – **Concrete operational**
AGE – 7-11 years approximately
CHARACTERISATION – Can think logically about objects and events.
Can appreciate numbers, weight, size and opposites at the same time, e.g. longer, shorter.

STAGE – **Formal operational**
AGE – 12 years plus approximately
CHARACTERISATION – Thinks logically about abstract propositions and can speculate.
Becomes concerned about hypothetical situations and the future.
Able to reflect on own thoughts.

3

Conception to birth

HUMAN REPRODUCTION

Our existence depends on the sexual relationship of two parents, mother and father. The organs in the human body which allow the species to continue are called the **reproductive organs**. These organs contain the cells which are programmed to start a new life (see Figure 3).

THE OVARIES AND THE TESTES

The cells which produce the 'seeds' which the male contributes to the formation of a new life are contained in the **testes** (singular: testis). The testes produce billions of male seeds but only one is necessary to start a new life. The seeds are called **spermatozoa**, sperm for short, and when they are released they swim about in a special fluid called

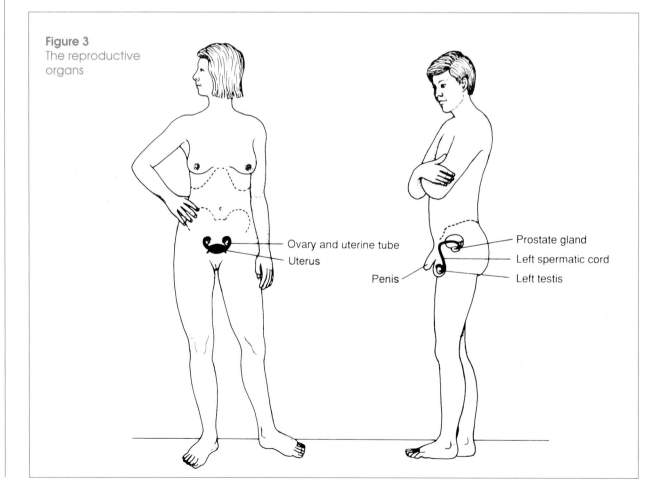

Figure 3
The reproductive organs

Ovary and uterine tube
Uterus

Prostate gland
Left spermatic cord
Penis
Left testis

seminal fluid which is made in a gland situated beside the testes.

The female pattern of seed production is different. The birthplace of the female seeds is in the **ovaries**. These seeds are called **ova** collectively and one seed is called an **ovum**. In the reproductive phase of a young woman's life, she has the potential for producing somewhere in the region of 200 000 ova. Some of these become mature ova and are released during the female **menstrual cycle**. Others never mature – they degenerate (decline) and die.

In the female, the production of mature ova is linked to the menstrual cycle. The menstrual cycle takes about 28 days to complete but this varies considerably from one individual to another. If fertilisation does not occur, the cycle ends in menstruation and the lining of the uterus is shed and discharged (during the menstrual period). **Hormones**, substances made in specialised glands in the body, are chemical messengers which control the whole process; oestrogen and progesterone are two such hormones.

CELL REPRODUCTION

The ability to form a new cell is based on information carried in a 'computer centre' in the cell **nucleus**. This contains chemical components and the most important one for cell reproduction is called **deoxyribonucleic acid (DNA)**. The particular configuration of the DNA molecules at the time of cell division determines the characteristic features transferred to the new cell.

Throughout life cells develop, mature and die so it is important that they can be reproduced in order to maintain life. Nerve cells are one exception. We are born with a supply of nerve cells and, in fact, we have many more than we need or ever use. Those which are not activated die off; also, in the decline phase of human development, many nerve cells degenerate and die. We will look at this in more detail in Chapter 9.

GENES AND CHROMOSOMES

The information necessary to reproduce a cell is held on thousands of tiny beads called **genes** which can either be dominant or recessive. The dominant gene is likely to have a greater influence. The genes are situated on strand-like structures called **chromosomes**.

Whenever a cell is about to reproduce, the chromosomes make an identical copy and so appear in pairs (see Figure 4). Each cell has 46 chromosomes or 23 pairs of chromosomes. Each

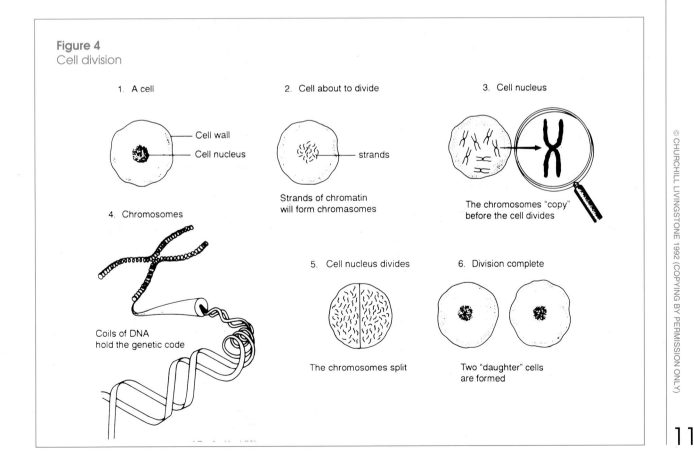

Figure 4
Cell division

1. A cell
   Cell wall
   Cell nucleus

2. Cell about to divide
   strands
   Strands of chromatin will form chromasomes

3. Cell nucleus
   The chromosomes "copy" before the cell divides

4. Chromosomes
   Coils of DNA hold the genetic code

5. Cell nucleus divides
   The chromosomes split

6. Division complete
   Two "daughter" cells are formed

© CHURCHILL LIVINGSTONE 1992 (COPYING BY PERMISSION ONLY)

of the 22 chromosome pairs carry thousands of genes which are coded and work together to complete all the internal structures and external appearance of each new life. The 23rd pair, in addition to contributing to bodily structure, is involved in determining the sex of the new being; that is, they consist of an 'X' (representing femaleness) or a 'Y' (representing maleness). The female can only contribute an X chromosome; the male produces both X and Y chromosomes, so his contribution can be either one or the other. The ovum and sperm each contribute half of the total chromosomes to the fertilised egg. The inherited differences between members of the same family are due to minute structural differences in parts of the chromosomes.

Now try Exercise 6.

● ●

EXERCISE 6

'The king divorced his wife, the queen, because she could not bear him a son and heir.'

Was there any justice in the king's actions? Give a logical reason for your answer based on what you have learned so far in this chapter.

(Answers on page 47)

● ●

FERTILISATION AND CONCEPTION

Stop and think about the wonder of human reproduction. Think of the millions of babies born in the world every day who are healthy, normal individuals. However, sometimes, for whatever reason, errors occur in the development process. Often, these are errors in genetic programming and are obvious at birth, for example, babies born with Down's syndrome. Other errors are less obvious and can only be detected by very careful cell studies; some remain undiscovered.

Fertilisation is the term given to the penetration of the ova by the male sperm which usually takes place in the fallopian, or uterine, tube. Each of the partners contributes half of the total chromosomal complement, that is, 22, plus one sex chromosome, so that the new being will have a total of 46 chromosomes.

The first stage of reproduction is when a sperm and ova, which have developed in the respective testes and ovary, are joined together in the female body. This process is called **conception** and can be defined as the moment a new life begins, when the two cells become joined together as one new cell.

See Exercise 7.

● ●

EXERCISE 7

Find a diagram which shows you how and where fertilisation takes place.

- How does the sperm manage to get access to the ova to complete the process of fertilisation?
- Where does the process of fertilisation take place in the female body?
- Where does the fertilised egg start growing and developing?
- What happens to an ovum if fertilisation does not occur?
- When is fertilisation most likely to be successful?

You might like to try and work out for yourself, or find out about, possible causes of infertility.

(Answers on page 47)

● ●

Once the complete set of instructions for the creation of a new life is in place, the process that follows is one of 'body building'. One cell divides into two, two into four, four into eight and so on. This process continues throughout life in order to maintain the body cells necessary for living, with the exception of the nerve cells.

From the moment successful fertilisation occurs the woman can be described as pregnant. However, the signs and symptoms of pregnancy are not usually apparent until after the first period is missed. It is at this stage that the mother seeks confirmation of her pregnancy, probably by consulting her general practitioner. It is possible, however, to carry out a pregnancy test without going to a doctor.

GESTATION PERIOD

The **gestation** period, that is, the term of a pregnancy, is 40 weeks in a human. Often the alternative (9 months) is referred to by the lay person. As the number of days and weeks in a month varies, a more accurate record can be obtained by selecting weeks as the time measurement.

Pregnancy is associated with dramatic physical changes, not only in the developing 'new life' but also in the mother's body – there is a partnership between the developing being and the mother.

In order to study the growth patterns that occur over the 40-week period more carefully many scientists divide this whole period into three sections, or phases: (See Figure 5)

• The **germinal** period – this covers the period from conception to implantation of the fertilised cell in the womb. It is during this period of cell division and cell specialisation that the whole foundation for body structure and function is determined.

• The **embryonic** period – this follows the development of the new life from the time of implantation to the stage when primitive development of the major structures of the body are evident at about 8-10 weeks. The fetal heart, for example, can be detected using electronic ultrasonic equipment. Once the major human structures are designed and in place, growth and functional development can proceed. The embryo is now known as the fetus.

• The **fetal** growth period – this begins with the transition from embryo to fetus at about 10 weeks until the baby is able to exist outside the mother's body.

Look again at Figure 5. Do you recognise the direction of development of the fetus? It goes from head to tail, and from the midline out to the periphery (the tips of the fingers).

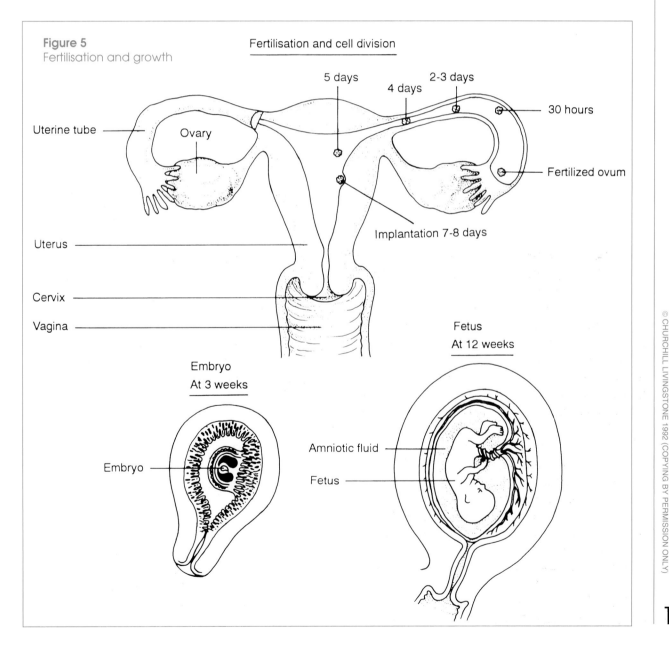

Figure 5
Fertilisation and growth

Fertilisation and cell division

5 days · 4 days · 2-3 days · 30 hours

Uterine tube · Ovary · Fertilized ovum

Implantation 7-8 days

Uterus

Cervix

Vagina

Fetus At 12 weeks

Embryo At 3 weeks

Embryo

Amniotic fluid

Fetus

13

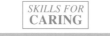
DEFECTIVE CHROMOSOMES

These are often unpredictable. Some change occurs in the copying process at the stage of cell division, when the germ (first) cells are being produced, and the result is that the chromosomes are not an exact copy of the originals. The consequences of this can be so severe that development cannot proceed and the products of conception are expelled, for example, in early abortions. With modern methods of detection it is often possible to detect such errors in the pre-birth or prenatal period.

See Exercise 8.

● ●

EXERCISE 8

Here are the results of some genetic and developmental errors:

• sickle-cell anaemia
• Down's syndrome
• haemophilia
• spina bifida.

You might like to investigate:

– what defect gives rise to the developmental disorder?
– how do these disorders affect the process of development?
– what, if anything, can be done to assist a better prognosis (that is, forecast for future progress) for each individual affected?

(Answers on page 47)

● ●

The developing fetus is extremely vulnerable so it is important that it is protected from such things as harmful organisms and poisonous substances. While the placenta prevents transfer of many germs some viruses can gain access and cause serious damage. The placenta is highly selective but some of the harmful substances contained in many drugs can cross the barrier and cause serious interference to the process of development. Therefore, all drugs should be regarded as potentially dangerous and avoided, except by medical prescription.

Examples of known, dangerous substances are alcohol, heroin, and nicotine but many are probably still unknown. Even dietary additives and other dietary substances are thought to have a harmful effect on development.

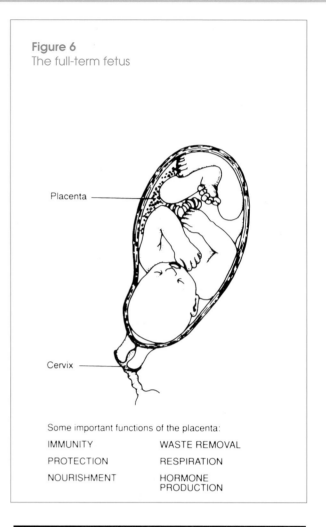

Figure 6
The full-term fetus

Placenta

Cervix

Some important functions of the placenta:

IMMUNITY	WASTE REMOVAL
PROTECTION	RESPIRATION
NOURISHMENT	HORMONE PRODUCTION

MONITORING OF FETAL DEVELOPMENT

• **Routine tests**
Testing the mother's blood and urine can indicate if the pregnancy is progressing normally.

• **External palpation of the abdomen**
As the fetus develops its different parts can be felt with careful palpation (that is, using the hands and fingers) of the mother's abdomen. This gives some useful information about the size and position of the fetus.

• **Internal examination**
This may be carried out at the first visit to the doctor or the clinic to assess the size and shape of the mother's pelvis, but it is rarely carried out as the pregnancy advances. It is very helpful as labour progresses.

• **Ultrasound scan**
The radiation from X-rays can have damaging effects so sound waves are used instead for a scan. By directing an instrument over the mother's abdomen and pelvis, the sound waves meet bone and soft tissue which vary in density. These parts

are represented by a picture on a screen and give valuable information about fetal progress without any obvious harm to the fetus.

• **Amniocentesis**

This is a procedure used to detect specific developmental abnormalities. Generally, it is confined to those women where there is a family history of defects in development, to older women or by special request. By examination of a specimen of the amniotic fluid – the fluid which surrounds and cushions the developing fetus in the womb – two important investigations are possible. If there is a raised level of the substance alphafetoprotein, it indicates there may be abnormalities such as anencephaly (failure of the brain to develop) which is not compatible with life, that is, the baby dies at or shortly after birth, or spina bifida (failure of the spinal canal to close properly). Other conditions, such as Down's syndrome, haemophilia or muscular dystrophy, can be detected early by chromosomal analysis of cells in the amniotic fluid. Normally, the test is performed between the 15th and 17th week. There is a slight risk of miscarriage (about 1%) so the reasons for carrying out the procedure are usually well justified. Another procedure is also used to detect abnormalities in the very early weeks of pregnancy, where a specimen of the developing placenta is obtained; this is called chorionic villus sampling (CVS).

Try Exercise 9.

● ●

EXERCISE 9

Find out more about pregnancy and from your research make a list of all the changes that take place in the mother's body during:

- weeks 1-14
- weeks 15-28
- weeks 29-40

(Answers on page 47)

● ●

LABOUR

This is a normal process which, hopefully, ends in the expulsion of a healthy, live baby at term or forty weeks. Should anything interfere with this normal process, however, it can have adverse effects on the mother, or the child, or both. For example, if the mother goes into premature labour

the fetus is also pre-term and therefore more vulnerable to problems such as birth asphyxia, which can cause cerebral palsy and other problems of prematurity.

There are relatively few incidences of birth injuries in modern times in the well-developed countries.

Continue your research in Exercise 10.

● ●

EXERCISE 10

Find out about the process of labour:

- What is labour?
- How do you recognise it has started?
- How long does it take?
- What are the different stages?

(Answers on page 47)

● ●

INFLUENCES ON FETAL DEVELOPMENT

Faults can occur in the development process which may affect the developmental process adversely, or halt further development at different stages during the process. Some of the possible causes for these faults are diet and drugs.

DIET

A pregnant woman requires a diet of approximately 2700 calories per day to meet the needs of herself and the fetus. The diet must be well-balanced to contain all the essential nutrients in the correct proportion. These nutrients are proteins, fats, carbohydrates, vitamins and minerals.

DRUGS

Probably one of the commonest drugs which adversely influence fetal development is the drug alcohol. The effects of alcohol on fetal development depend to a large extent on how much alcohol is consumed. However, as little as two glasses of wine taken by the pregnant mother per day, on a regular basis, may be enough to put the fetus at risk.

Drug addicts may transfer their addiction to the unborn fetus. This threatens the survival of the newborn, who may die from prematurity or the consequence of respiratory disease. These babies may also suffer serious withdrawal symptoms if they are not given appropriate treatment after birth. Even with treatment they may subsequently present symptoms of cerebral or brain irritation, such as irritability, disturbed sleep patterns and lack of fine muscle control.

All drugs should be considered potentially harmful if taken during pregnancy. It is unwise and unsafe for an expectant mother to take any drug, even if it seems harmless and is readily available, because the side effects on the fetus may not be known.

Drugs such as antibiotics (used to treat infections), tranquillisers (given to reduce anxiety), anticoagulants (which prevent clotting of the blood) and anticonvulsants (administered to control fits) are a few examples of the kinds of prescribed drugs which must be carefully checked by medical practitioners if taken during pregnancy.

Smoking is a drug because it contains an addictive substance called nicotine. Smoking is a serious danger to health in general terms but the main effect on the developing fetus if the mother smokes during pregnancy is 'oxygen starvation'. The oxygen in the circulating blood is replaced by carbon monoxide, so starving the fetus of essential oxygen. This can result in prematurity (birth before full term) or low birth weight. The incidence of miscarriage and stillbirth also seems to be higher if the mother smokes.

INFECTIONS AND OTHER DISEASES

Already, we have discovered that some harmful organisms can get across the placental barrier. The effects can be harmful, either during the period of fetal development or after the birth of the baby. We will look at some of the more common examples but you may want to explore others in your own time.

RUBELLA

If a mother contracts rubella during the first 12 weeks of pregnancy, the consequences can be disastrous. As high as 50% of fetuses will have developmental defects of one kind or another. The common defects include congenital (i.e. born with) heart disease, blindness caused by cataract formation (a film growing over the lens), deafness, and mental retardation (failure of the brain to develop completely, to varying degrees).

Thankfully, the incidence of the disease has been controlled to a considerable extent by the development of a vaccine and by the availability of tests to determine whether or not the pregnant mother has been infected or is immune.

HEPATITIS B

If a mother is infected by this virus, she is likely to transmit the disease to her unborn baby. Drug users who inject drugs into their veins, especially if they share dirty needles, are particularly at risk from hepatitis B.

HUMAN IMMUNE-DEFICIENCY VIRUS (HIV)

If a pregnant woman has been exposed to this virus, for example, through sexual intercourse, transfusions or needle-sharing, and is infected, she may deliver a baby at risk of being or becoming HIV positive.

DIABETES

While many mothers who are known diabetics do, and are encouraged to, have a family, particular care is required during the pregnancy. Babies of these mothers tend, if not carefully supervised during the fetal period, to become grossly overweight during the later months and this can cause extra strain on vital organs like the heart.

PSYCHOSOCIAL AND COGNITIVE DEVELOPMENT

Behaviour occurs before birth because the fetus moves and responds to sound and touch. From the moment of conception the nature versus nurture influences are at work.

The internal environment of the mother's body influences the fertilised egg and its genetic inheritance. The mother's health, or lack of it, affects the developing baby's growth and development. What she eats, drinks or smokes, and any viruses she contracts, can have an adverse effect on her unborn child. The fetus is totally dependent on the mother's psychosocial health for its well-being, and this interaction can never be separated. Her reaction to being pregnant, and her lifestyle, influences the developing baby.

MATERNAL EMOTIONS

Despite the fact that there are no direct connections between the maternal and fetal nervous systems, the mother's emotional state can influence fetal reactions and development. Emotions bring the mother's autonomic (independent) nervous system into action, and certain chemicals and hormones are released into the bloodstream. These substances cross the placenta and enter the fetal circulation causing irritation to the fetus. Some studies have shown a marked increase in fetal movements in emotionally stressed mothers.

If the mother's stress lasts for several weeks, fetal activity may continue at an exaggerated level. In brief upsets, heightened activity generally settles down again.

One result of prolonged maternal distress, whether from partnership difficulties, negative feelings towards the baby or catastrophic life events, is a low-birth-weight or premature baby.

Usually, the more relaxed a mother is during normal labour and delivery, the easier and shorter the process of giving birth will be. Highly anxious mothers, who are sensitive to pain and fearful of the birth process, tend to have more difficult deliveries and more irritable babies. It is known that there is a greater incidence of behaviour disorders and chronic illness in children of mothers stressed during pregnancy. The same stress may be present postnatally and may affect the baby's psychosocial development.

BIRTH AND BONDING

Birth should be a joyful experience, with a happy relaxed mother supported by her husband or partner sharing the experience with her.

The care of the newborn infant is exacting and tiring. Many social and emotional forces combine to motivate parents in tackling the task. The process of attachment, or bonding, between parents and baby begins as soon as pregnancy is recognised and is particularly powerful around the time of birth. Most new parents look at their newly born baby and exclaim how beautiful he or she is, although to the birth attendants the baby may be anything but beautiful!

These first few moments of life are of crucial importance and, if the baby is not in need of immediate medical attention, he is warmly wrapped and given to the parents to hold, touch, admire and examine. This sensory stimulation is a two-way process. Breast feeding in these early moments helps increase the emotional and sensory stimulation.

Shortly after birth, the infant is often quiet, alert and receptive and eye-to-eye contact is established with his parents. It is almost as if this behaviour is pre-programmed and designed for the bonding process. Separation of mother and baby at this time has been associated with the occurrence of less desirable handling practices many weeks later and an increased risk of child abuse. Obviously, the majority of mothers and babies tolerate disruption of the bonding process if a medical emergency arises, and no ill effects result from this. It is the immature, stressed mother with mixed feelings towards her situation who is most likely to be vulnerable to separation from her baby at this crucial time.

Find out more about birth by doing Exercise 11.

• •

EXERCISE 11

Discuss with other people different experiences they have had, or heard about, with regard to:

- place of confinement
- amount of technology used, e.g. forceps, Caesarian section.

• •

4

Infancy

PHYSICAL DEVELOPMENT

THE NEWBORN

During the first year of life dramatic changes take place.

GENERAL FEATURES

The average newborn baby weighs about 3.5 kilograms (7½ pounds) and is approximately 50 centimetres (20 inches) long. Babies can vary in size, and still be within the normal limits, depending on the genetic information transferred from the parents. The circumference of the head measures about 35 centimetres (14 inches). This is an important measurement in case the head size increases abnormally, as happens, for example, with hydrocephalus, a disorder of the fluid circulation round the brain.

The baby's **skin** is covered by variable amounts of vernix, a cheese like substance, and lanugo, or fine hair, produced in fetal life. Some babies have different kinds of red, blue or blue-black birthmarks. Most of these are harmless and will eventually disappear.

Jaundice is a common feature in the newborn and may take a day or so to appear. It shows as a yellowing of the skin, and sometimes the whites of the eyes, and varies in severity. If unresolved it can have serious consequences, for example, brain damage. It is usually caused by the breakdown of unrequired red blood cells once the baby can breathe in sufficient quantities of oxygen. The pigment from the broken-down blood cells cannot be eliminated efficiently by the relatively immature kidney system, so it circulates round in the bloodstream for a few days until the kidneys have successfully got rid of it.

The skin of the baby's hands and feet often appears almost blue in colour while the rest of the skin looks quite pink. Although the circulation is still immature, if the lips or tongue appear unusually blue there could be an underlying lung or heart disorder interfering with the oxygenation of the blood.

The **abdomen** appears large in proportion to the chest; the remnant of the umbilical cord still attached drops off in about a week.

The **eyes** appear blue-grey in most babies at first, except perhaps in dark skinned babies. The final colour may not be determined for 2-3 months. During the first weeks it is quite common for a newborn (or 'neonate') to squint when he opens his eyes and tries to focus. While this is perfectly normal it should correct itself within the first 6 months. The eyes should be clear and free from any sticky material. The ears are often flattened and covered with fine hair.

The **tongue** may have tiny white spots on its surface; this is perfectly normal, unless the spots change character and appear like a persistent coating.

ASSESSMENT

Assessment of the baby at birth is important, both to exclude any defects and to provide a basis from which further development can be predicted and assessed. Various tests have been developed to rate the baby's physical state and these are referred to as **rating scales.**

The **Apgar score** is based on an assessment of the vital functions at birth and again 5 minutes after birth. A normal, healthy baby with a maximum score of 10 would cry vigorously (so using his lungs), appear pink in colour, have a heart rate of over 100, use his limbs actively (good muscle tone) and have the normal reflexes present. If a baby falls below a score of four this indicates that he may not survive unless he receives immediate medical attention.

Reflexes are responses to stimuli without the voluntary control of the brain. Apart from the protective function of some reflex actions, other reflex actions will only give an indication that the nervous system is functioning normally. Some other reflexes are tested but it is not clear what the significance of the findings are except that they are present in normal, healthy babies.

Reflex tests act as a basis for assessment of nervous system function. Examples of such reflexes are the Moro reflex, the Babinski reflex, and the Rooting reflex. Try to find out more about these and other reflexes of the newborn.

Apart from establishing that the baby is structurally and functionally normal, a record of the detailed examination of the newborn provides an important base from which to determine progress. For example, soon after birth baby's length and body weight are recorded. Other important observations are made, such as head circumference, heart and lung function, and examination of mouth, limbs, skin and genital areas. These observations are significant because a deformity or malfunction can have detrimental effects on the development process. However, with modern surgical techniques and safer anaesthesia, many abnormalities detected in the newborn can be corrected soon after birth, for example, cleft palate and heart defects.

THE FIRST YEAR

Immense changes take place during the first year of the baby's life. If you were able to compare the skeletal X-ray of the baby with that of the adult you would be able to recognise the growth that has taken place in the skeletal framework, that is, the length of the long bones, the density of the bones and the final formation of the heads of the bones within the joint spaces.

Compared with the newborn of other animals, such as dogs, cats, cows and sheep, the human baby is rather immature. Do you know of any newborn baby that can stand and run about soon after birth? Newborn babies are totally dependent on help from carers (especially parents) to survive and acquire the complex knowledge and skills which will help them function as competent adults in later life.

THE NEONATE

'Neonate' is the term used to describe the newborn baby up to the age of around 1 month. During this early period the tiny infant has rather a tenuous grip on the world he has entered. He is uncoordinated, sleeps most of the time and during his waking periods spends most of his time taking in food.

THE INFANT

The term 'infant' refers to the baby during his first year of life. Physical progress during this period is dramatic and on page 7 we used the term milestones which are the 'measuring guides' used to assess the normal development process.
See Exercise 12.

• •

EXERCISE 12

Below is a section from a growth and development chart. Put together a chart of your own which includes all 4 areas of development – Posture and large motor skills, Vision and fine motor skills, Hearing and language, Social behaviour and play. You can enter milestones of development on the chart from your own experience with a young baby or from your reading. Some examples have been shown to get you started.

(Answers – completed chart on page 48)

DEVELOPMENT CHART

MONTHS	POSTURE AND LARGE MOTOR SKILLS	HEARING AND LANGUAGE
0		
1		
2		Social smiles
3		Coos or
4		gurgles
5		
6	Sits up with	
7	support	
8		
9		
10	Crawls or moves from spot	
11		
12		
13		
14		
15		
16		
17		
18		
Years		
2		
3		
4		
5		

PRINCIPLES OF DEVELOPMENT

We noticed that in fetal growth, the direction of growth is from head to toe and from the midline to the fingertips. All children follow a **sequential** pattern of development, that is, they hold up their heads before they sit up and stand before they can walk. These are called **non-variables** because they are the same in all children. However, the one variable is the *rate* of development, for example, some 1 year olds can walk, others cannot; some 6-month-old babies do not have any teeth but others have one, two or even four.

Development of skills depends on the further development of the brain and the nervous system. Bundles of nerve fibres, which carry messages to the brain for interpretation and response, become more highly developed giving the child more control over voluntary activity.

It is now widely accepted that the experiences of the first 2 years have a lasting influence on the growing child. Learning and emotion are closely dependent on each other. Given inborn potential for development and environmental opportunities, the infant needs motivation to learn and progress. The driving force of the will to learn has its roots in the quality of relationships given to the infant from birth.

BONDING, SECURITY AND PARENTING

The need for love and security, new experiences, praise, recognition and responsibility are as important to the infant as they are to the elderly. Love and security are achieved if the infant experiences, from birth onwards, a stable, continuous, dependable and loving relationship with his parents or care giver (who themselves enjoy a rewarding relationship with others). The healthy development of the personality, the ability to respond to affection and eventually become a loving, caring parent, depend on this relationship.

Security is established if there is a stable home where surroundings become familiar, attitudes and behaviour are consistent and a routine is established. This in turn provides the infant with the reassurance to explore his environment, to reach out, to crawl or walk, knowing that he will be comforted if his security is threatened.

'Parenting' is the term used to explain the ways in which behaviour is influenced by the parent's personality, together with the infant's characteristics and the social environment in which the parent-child relationship takes place. The infant's physical appearance, health and maturity may influence a parent's initial reaction and the bonding process. A premature baby, for example, is immature in everything, including his responses. Sometimes an infant's temperament may be difficult – different temperaments bring out different responses from the parents or care givers.

TRUST VERSUS MISTRUST

The young infant learns to express a greater variety of emotions as he develops trust and security. Abusive, inconsistent or neglectful parents foster a sense of mistrust and insecurity. Emotion expressed in the infant's early play indicates the development of the **sensorimotor skills**; the stimulation provided by toys and rattles can become an intensely absorbing experience. The infant gains control and coordination of his muscles and achieves his milestones. He enjoys praise and recognition of his achievement, even at the baby stage. These new experiences are all essential to learning processes.

COGNITIVE CHANGES

Compared to animals, the human infant is helpless at birth. He has over 48 primitive reflexes which enable him to breathe, suck, swallow, blink and grasp. During the first year of life many of these reflexes come under conscious control or disappear. These reflexes are used as an indicator of developmental progress.

SENSORY STIMULATION

The infant learns about his environment by the sensory stimulation of his five senses, sight, hearing, taste, touch and smell. He experiences hunger, heat, cold and pain from which he was protected before birth. His response to this is to become restless and start to cry. If a crying infant is picked up he normally quietens down, at least for a time, indicating his responsiveness to sensations of being held. Physical and psychological needs are so closely related that feeding and changing him to make him comfortable physically also improves his psychological well-being. Closeness, warmth, caressing and talking all provoke a response, even in a newly born baby.

The newly born baby sleeps approximately two-thirds of the day and is alert or drowsy the rest of the time. As the brain develops, so too do the centres in the brain which interpret the information received from the five senses. In this way, cognitive development is built up as the infant increases his ability to put together the sensory information necessary to make sense of his physical world. If these sensory experiences are impaired as, for example, in a blind baby, permanent changes are produced in the structure of the visual centre in the brain so that, even if sight is restored, visual input would be severely retarded.

Piaget's first stage of cognitive development, sensorimotor, describes how the newborn baby with simple reflexes achieves the knowledge of a 2-year-old child.

The infant becomes quite skilled at collecting information about his world from what he sees, hears, touches, tastes and smells. With a growth in motor skills, he gradually gains access to objects and people. Piaget subdivided the sensorimotor stage into substages (see below).

SENSORIMOTOR STAGE – SUBDIVISIONS

- FIRST MONTH (reflex stage)
  Response to all objects is the same
  e.g. sucks a piece of clothing as well
  as a nipple.

- SECOND MONTH
  Sleeps less. More responsive to
  environment:
  – becomes aware of objects and
  follows them, within his visual field
  – responds to different sounds
  Social smiling begins; if awake and alert
  will respond strongly when talked to,
  making vocal sounds in return.
  Crying now accompanied by tears.

- FOURTH TO EIGHTH MONTH
  Acquires hand and eye coordination:
  – reaches out for objects
  – learns about environment beyond his
  body
  By 8 months can anticipate events,
  e.g. knows when it is meal time, bed
  time.
  Looks for objects that disappear.
  Becomes distressed and crawls after
  mother when she leaves the room.

All this knowledge is absorbed and interacts with the infant's emotional and social development; from it he will develop his behaviour and actions.

SPEECH AND COMMUNICATION

From birth the infant gradually acquires and expands his range of sounds and gestures, the first of which is crying. From birth the infant hears the sounds of speech – when he hears speech he becomes still, looks around for the voice and opens his eyes wider. By the age of 2 months he makes cooing sounds that contain the basic sounds of all languages. The more stimulation the infant receives, the more he will vocalise. His response depends on his mother's responses, on her expressions of love and her tone of voice.

By the age of 6 months the infant produces only the sounds contained in the language he hears. During the second 6 months of life the infant learns to control his speech and use it for social interactions with people and toys. He begins to understand spoken words like 'no' and 'wave bye bye'.

We often use words to express ideas and silently spoken sentences to solve problems. How much our language ability influences our cognitive development is unclear. One study of deaf children who had not been taught sign language showed that their ability to solve problems was unaffected. Some psychologists dispute this and claim that language provides a rich vocabulary to help give meaning to ideas.
See Exercise 13.

● ●

EXERCISE 13

Think about an infant who is deprived of any of the 5 senses. What effect would this have on his cognitive development?

(Answers on page 47)

● ●

5

Childhood years

PHYSICAL DEVELOPMENT

THE TODDLER AND THE PRE-SCHOOL CHILD

During the first year of the child's life there is very rapid growth and development: the child goes from an uncoordinated being who requires total support to a more physically independent child.

During the next phase, growth slows down but development continues to advance. Bowel and bladder control increase as the internal muscles function more effectively. The muscles of the trunk and body develop allowing the child to jump,

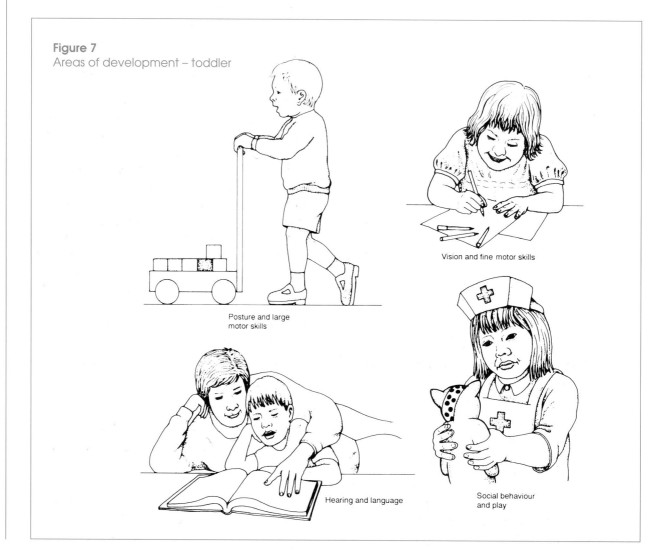

Figure 7
Areas of development – toddler

Posture and large
motor skills

Vision and fine motor skills

Hearing and language

Social behaviour
and play

climb, run and leap. He uses his arms to shake objects, pull toys and tug at things which get stuck. Balance has developed and the child learns to stand on one leg, walk steadily along a thin plank or kick a ball. Hair grows to replace fine baby hair and is longer and thicker in texture. The child is physically more able to provide for his needs, for example, he can feed himself, go to the toilet unaided and dress and undress most of his clothing. He can use a variety of toys which require fine manipulation and can turn pages of children's books. His manipulative skills enable him to carry out quite difficult tasks, like tying shoe laces and fastening buttons (see Figure 7).

Try Exercise 14 when you have time.

● ●

EXERCISE 14

Try to visit a playgroup or nursery, or (with the parents' knowledge), observe a group of 2, 3 and 4 year olds in your own neighbourhood.

Using the following headings, make a list of the skills developed by each of the age groups. You can add other relevant headings like 'rest' and 'sleep patterns'. You can also subdivide headings, such as play, into 'large motor movement' and 'fine motor movement using the hands and fingers'.

2 year olds: Child's name:

• Feeding • Dressing • Sleeping • Toileting
• Playing

Do the same with 3 year olds and 4 year olds. Three or four children in each group should give you enough information from which to draw conclusions.

● ●

PSYCHOSOCIAL AND COGNITIVE DEVELOPMENT

THE TODDLER

During the first year of life, the child acquires knowledge and ideas about the world in which he lives. He forms attachments with a small group of people – his immediate family and perhaps grandparents, childminders or care givers.

SPEECH AND COMMUNICATION

Learning to walk opens up a new world of exploration, constraints and restrictions. The toddler gains self-awareness and independence through these experiences. Play becomes increasingly important in his development as he experiments and works out simple tasks for himself. Piaget looked upon this stage as the beginning of problem solving – the end of the sensorimotor stage of development and the beginning of pre-operational thought symbolised by language, play and a world of make-believe (see page 9).

Hearing his own voice stimulates the toddler to repeat words. At first, he imitates the speech of others by saying single words. A continual stream of jargon, with recognisable words mixed in with it, comes before the stringing of words together into two-word sentences at about the time of his second birthday. At this time the child also learns to associate objects and people with their names, as he begins to comprehend his native language. Memory develops too, as he processes increasing amounts of information.

ACQUIRING SOCIAL SKILLS

As the child communicates his feelings and his self-esteem grows, so too does his desire to gain bowel and bladder control. Before the age of 18 months, the child's elimination processes are involuntary. Toilet training depends on the motivation to learn and the maturation of the sphincters (circular muscles) involved. The learning of this task is often a source of emotional conflict between parent and child. A full bladder and rectum cause an unpleasant feeling. The child gains pleasure from emptying his bowel and bladder, whether it is socially convenient or not! His acceptance of toilet training shows he wants to be like his parents and to obtain their approval and love. He also acquires other social skills, such as the use of cutlery to feed himself and suitable social behaviour.

SELF-IMAGE AND INDEPENDENCE

The child's self-image depends very much on the sense of trust which has grown out of a loving, caring relationship with his parents and care givers. He has learned to accept or rebel against certain patterns of behaviour. He knows not to touch or climb certain things and not to pull or knock over objects. During this time he must be reassured that if he goes beyond the limits of his mother's patience and makes her angry he will not lose her love. His self-image will be increased by what his mother communicates to him. Love, care, praise and attention develop his self-esteem. Failure to achieve this, and some measure of independence, can result in feelings of worthlessness, shame and doubt.

If the toddler is given plenty of opportunities to explore and practise tasks on his own, with adult support, he will emerge with a positive sense of his own worth. If not, when he is asked to do something he may rebel with a firm 'No!' or may have temper tantrums or breath-holding attacks.

THE PRE-SCHOOL CHILD (2-5 YEARS)

The pre-school years, ages 2-5, are a period of broadening horizons. The child, deeply attached to his parents, becomes increasingly influenced by brothers and sisters, extended family, nursery school teachers and his own peer group (or equals).

The child is now capable of thinking about an event and using symbols to represent it, for example, the Wendy house, dressing up or using a cardboard box as a car. In the same short period, from 2-7 years approximately, the child's vocabulary increases from two-word sentences to over 10,000 words and he masters the basic grammar of his native language.

SOCIALISATION AND PLAY

Socialisation is the process by which children acquire the behaviour, beliefs and motives that are valued by their family and cultural group. Parents train their children by rewarding responses they wish to strengthen and by punishing responses they wish to get rid of. The child also observes and identifies with others and develops the first signs of a conscience.

A secure child usually relates to others easily and quickly. A child who is overdependent and insecure often has difficulties in relating to others. Children who are over-disciplined by their parents may become withdrawn and unhappy. On the other hand, children who are given little or no discipline may become over-dependent and unhappy. Parents who show authority, and who reason with their children, are most likely to have children who are competent and friendly.

The home environment may change during this

time – the child may acquire brothers or sisters, or move house; the parents may divorce. A friendly, competent child is more likely to adjust to these changes. Brothers and sisters interact from infancy and compete for affection, attention and toys. They respond to each other and to other children socially, and anti-socially, by playing, hitting or fighting.

Learning to play with others is an important part of the socialising process. To begin with, children relate to others through fantasy and parallel play. Parallel play means that when three or four children are playing together in a Wendy House each one will be involved in his own fantasy world. Eventually, the child associates with others in his group and interactive play occurs – 'Cowboys and Indians' or 'Mummies and Daddies.' By school age, children begin to join in cooperative play where playthings are shared, games are organised and friends are made. Over-criticism of the child's play can lead to a sense of guilt.

The child also becomes aware of his sex through play. Gender-appropriate behaviour occurs. Put very simply this means little girls dress up and little boys play war games. This behaviour is reinforced by parents, family and nursery school teachers. (See *Skills for Caring – Clients as Individuals* for a more detailed look at the subject of gender.)

PHYSICAL DEVELOPMENT

THE SCHOOL CHILD (5-10 YEARS)

During this period physical changes are less obvious although growth and development are continuing.

One of the striking characteristic features of this age group is the loss of baby teeth. This is a natural biological process. Milk teeth are designed to meet the needs of the infant and toddler. Eventually, they are no longer strong enough to cope with foodstuffs which require to be mechanically chopped up and chewed in the mouth before they enter the digestive process. Even in fetal life preparation for this change has occurred: the tooth buds develop in the jaws and gums so that when they are needed they push out and replace the milk teeth.

MATURATION

This period in the growing child's life is one of **maturation**. In other words, as well as a continual increase in body size, and changes in body shape, a development process takes place because the brain cells are becoming more sophisticated and specialised. The brain begins to function more obviously as a processing unit, that is, there are more refined interconnections between the parts of the brain; this is what makes the human being superior to lesser animals in judgement, reasoning, analysis and decision-making. For example, a child of 5 is more likely to recognise and avoid dangerous situations than a 2 year old.

This process of maturation is closely linked to development potential because, as well as the hereditary factors which predict the future adult, the experiences that the growing child has as he interacts with his environment also enable him to develop the advanced physical skills associated with this age group. These build on the earlier preliminary skills, such as coordination. Advanced skills include whole body development, like skipping or riding a bicycle, as well as the specific refinements of hand function required in writing, painting and drawing. Obviously, the more opportunity there is for the child to experience different activities the more skilled he is likely to become.

The child's physical growth depends on other factors too, like diet, sleep, a safe environment and protection from illness and injury. You may remember contracting many of the common infectious diseases, like mumps, chicken-pox and measles, when you were a child. You would also have been protected from others, such as polio, by being immunised in early childhood, with further protection later from 'booster' injections.

Growth in childhood is not predictable. If you look at a group of 5-8 year olds you will find that they vary in height and weight. A child of 6 years may be around 105 centimetres (3½ feet) tall and about 22½ kilograms (50 pounds) in weight; by the time that child reaches adolescence he will be nearer 1½ metres (5 feet) tall and around 45 kilograms (100 pounds) in weight. Also, growth occurs at different rates in individuals. Boys between the ages of 5 and 10 years tend to be slightly heavier and stronger than girls. The development of the muscles and growth of bones alter the shape of the body; 'baby fat' disappears and the child's physical inherited characteristics are more obvious. It is now easy to see, for example, that a child has his father's nose and his mother's eye colour.
See Exercise 15.

• •

EXERCISE 15

- It might be fun to find an old family album and try to identify the young people in the photographs. How many can you name correctly?
- You may be able to make some interesting observations about development and heredity.

• •

ACQUIRING SKILLS

As children grow, their physical skills develop but at different rates and at different times. This is related to the experiences they have. For example, if we take two 5 year olds, the first one may be able to swim and the second cannot, but the second may well be able to ride a bicycle while the first cannot. Complex skills need practice to make perfect. However, a skill cannot be learned if the brain and body systems have not developed to the required level. You can try encouraging a 7-month-old child to walk by taking him by both hands; you are unlikely to succeed in making him walk independently because his body has not developed sufficiently for him to support his weight and his balance is still immature.

As the child develops physically he becomes more agile; he has more power to sustain activity, is stronger and has greater coordination. Many parents describe the energy of their young children as inexhaustible! However, activity has to be balanced with adequate sleep so that the 'batteries are recharged' ready for more activity. If this doesn't happen, then muscles overtire; muscle tiredness can lead to problems like 'proneness to accidents or injury' and make the child more vulnerable to disease.

Skills-acquisition helps the child to gain independence and to respond to the environment in which he lives; he can increase his learning because he has increased his ability to explore and take part in things, both alone and with others.
Try Exercise 16.

● ●

EXERCISE 16

Think back to your days as a youngster and try to remember when you first achieved the following:

- swimming a breadth of the swimming pool
- riding a bicycle
- playing tennis
- painting a picture
- drawing a face
- climbing a ladder
- climbing a tree
- taking part in a treasure hunt
- orienteering
- scoring a goal in a ball game.

If none of these fits your lifestyle, make up your own list.

Once you have completed your list, ask a friend or relative to list the activities in the order in which *they* achieved them. You will probably find striking variations.

● ●

What can you conclude from the results of Exercise 16?

PSYCHOSOCIAL AND COGNITIVE DEVELOPMENT

THE SCHOOL CHILD – (5-10 YEARS)

Going to school is an important new experience but a child may have been prepared for it by nursery education. At nursery the child learns to spend part of the day away from his mother, in unfamiliar surroundings, with unfamiliar adults for whose attention he has to compete. During this time he also learns to compete with, and compare himself to, his peers.

School is a way of life from 5-16 years of age, whatever the child's ability, intellect or social class.

A child's integration into the school system, and his progress, depend to a large extent on his ability to express himself. There are wide social class differences in language development. Children who are encouraged to hold conversations and who have stories and nursery rhymes as part of their daily routine (similar to the school system), tend to gain more from their schooling than other less stimulated children. Imagine the effect poor language development might have on a child's schooling. His progress will be delayed if he has difficulty expressing himself clearly, asking questions and grasping new ideas. He may also be rejected by his peers.

In the early years most schools are discovery orientated. Most children adapt well if their attention and natural curiosity are captured.

At about 6 or 7 years of age children undergo a remarkable change in their ability to understand and think – gone is the fantasy world of make-believe play. This is the period of concrete operations described by Piaget, that is, logical reasoning about concrete things.

Teachers' attitudes, values and beliefs increasingly affect the child. They may be different to those learned in the home and may lead to emotional conflict, lowered self-esteem and learning difficulties. To succeed at school the child needs to resolve and adapt to the environment outside the home.

Children with lowered self-esteem are likely to be anxious and insecure. Childhood fears and anxieties show themselves in many ways through nightmares, sleep disturbances, bedwetting, fears, phobias, obsessions, tics, stealing, vandalism or truancy. Imposing standards of behaviour that are too high or inconsistent will make the problem worse. Like-minded children may gang up and indulge in bullying and teasing others.

At this age, learning and observing the behaviour of parents, brothers and sisters, teachers and peers are of great importance when acquiring moral judgement and acceptable social behaviour. Behaviour is reinforced by 'the gang'. The gang is usually single sex and is important in and out of school in Cubs, Brownies, sports clubs or dancing classes where common interests are shared.

6

Adolescence

PHYSICAL DEVELOPMENT

The period of time between childhood or adulthood is called **adolescence**. It is not the same thing as **puberty.**

PUBERTY

Puberty is the term used to describe the biological changes which take place in the body and which transform the boy or girl from an immature being to a mature man or woman capable of sexual reproduction. This requires major changes involving the sex organs within each reproductive system in the male and the female. These changes are brought about by the production of hormones, governed by the master gland situated in the brain called the pituitary gland.

The pituitary gland conducts the 'orchestra' of other glands in the body; the glands related to puberty are the ovaries and the testes. The message to the pituitary gland to orchestrate hormone production from these glands comes from a control centre situated deep in the brain substance. First of all, the pituitary gland increases production of its own growth hormones and produces other hormones, which in turn instruct the ovaries and testes to begin the process of producing ripe ova and sperm, the seeds necessary for fertilisation and germination. Once started, this process continues in a regular pattern formation during adult life.

Puberty therefore marks the beginning of adolescence and is clearly seen when a young girl starts her first menstrual period. A young boy starts to have erections of his penis and is able to ejaculate, that is, to release seminal fluid which contains sperm.

ADOLESCENCE

It is more difficult to define exactly when adolescence starts and ends. This is because it includes all the changes which are taking place in the body which lead to puberty *and* all the changes which occur after puberty until adulthood is reached.
Try Exercise 17.

EXERCISE 17

If you have (or can borrow) a class photograph from school (when you were about 12 or 13 years of age) take a look at the girls in the group, then glance at the boys. What observations can you make?

DEVELOPMENT OF SECONDARY CHARACTERISTICS

BREAST DEVELOPMENT

One of the early signs of puberty in the female is the development of the breasts. You may have seen some girls in your class photograph who have obvious 'busts' while others are less developed. This development is in preparation for the breasts or mammary glands to produce milk, the process of lactation, in order to feed the offspring. As the adolescent female's menstrual cycle becomes established, she may experience temporary fullness of her breasts, often accompanied by tingling sensations prior to menstruation. Had she conceived and pregnancy begun this process would have

© CHURCHILL LIVINGSTONE 1992 (COPYING BY PERMISSION ONLY)

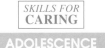

continued and her breasts would eventually have produced milk. The breasts have varying amounts of fatty tissue from one female to another, so the size does not necessarily determine the degree of glandular function.

AXILLARY AND PUBIC HAIR

Both sexes develop hair in the pubic area. In boys it may be an early sign of puberty but often appears later than in girls. Initially, it may be quite sparse and thickens towards the end of adolescence or in early adulthood. Underarm hair generally appears after pubic hair and may be 1 or 2 years later; the appearance of axillary hair before pubic hair is not abnormal but is more unusual. Boys also develop facial hair which becomes the beard area. This is also sparse at first, giving rise to the question 'to shave or not to shave?'! Some boys and girls have the added nuisance of acne. Because a male does not have any hair on his chest it does not mean he is 'weak': some males never develop any significant chest hair, but if they do it usually appears in late adolescence or adulthood.

DEVELOPMENT OF TESTES AND SCROTUM

As well as developing pubic hair, a young adolescent boy's testes enlarge. These are housed in the scrotum and its increasing size soon becomes obvious. The skin of the scrotum changes character, becoming thicker in texture and redder in colour. This is followed by growth of the penis which is part of a general body growth spurt. Once this development has occurred, the young adolescent male is capable of ejaculation and may have his first experience of a sudden erection of his penis, with release of seminal fluid, during sleep.

DEVELOPMENT OF THE UTERUS AND OVARIES

Although it cannot be seen in the young female her uterus increases in size with the production of hormones and this allows **ovulation** to occur. Ovulation is the release of a ripe ovum from the ovary each 28 days approximately. The linings of the vagina become thicker, more sensitive, moist and vascular (supplied with blood vessels) in preparation for successful intercourse.

There is no specified normal time for the girl to have her first menstrual period, but it usually occurs somewhere between 10 and 14 years of age and on average during the 12th year. In some girls it occurs quite normally later in adolescence.

GROWTH SPURT

The onset of puberty is also associated with an obvious growth spurt. This is due to the increase in production of the growth hormone as glandular activity speeds up. It is the most rapid growth period in both boys and girls since early childhood and can add approximately 6-9 inches (15-22 centimetres) to the height of girls and boys in a space of about 3 years. Generally, boys grow taller than girls. Also, the shape of the body changes due to marked muscular development and there is now a noticeable difference in physical strength between the male and female sex.

The direction of growth may not be as clearly 'head to toe' as in early childhood. Some boys and girls become long and lanky and appear to be all legs. Boys wearing long trousers instead of shorts need to have them replaced not just because of wear and tear but also because they 'grow out of them'. Girls become more shapely, that is, as well as the rounded contour of the chest due to breast development there is also a rounding of the hips so that they differ in shape from their male counterpart who tends to retain more slender hips. However, boys develop broader shoulders and chests as the large skeletal muscles develop. The growth of the skull is less obvious. This is not due to increased brain size (as many young adolescents would like to think!) but to a thickening of the bones of the skull.

VOICE CHANGES IN THE MALE

Before the onset of puberty the larynx, the organ which houses the vocal cords necessary for voice production, is very similar in both male and female. For example, many young choir boys have a true soprano voice as good as their female counterparts. As other changes occur in the body at the onset of puberty so changes occur in the male larynx. It becomes noticeably enlarged due to an increase in the size of the cartilaginous structures and forms what we call the Adam's apple, a projection of enlarged cartilage (a strong elastic substance) at the front of the throat. This development affects voice production, which lowers or deepens in tone so high-pitched sounds cannot be produced. The process takes some time to complete, years rather than months, and the unpredictable sound that emerges during this biological change is often referred to as 'the voice breaking'.

PSYCHOSOCIAL AND COGNITIVE DEVELOPMENT

Adolescence is a period of change – physical, sexual, social and psychological. It is likely to be a challenging and sometimes difficult stage in a young person's struggle towards maturity as well as a period of high hopes, new experiences and expanding opportunities.

A few generations ago adolescence as we know it today was non-existent. Many teenagers worked a 14-hour day and moved from childhood to adulthood with virtually no transition. Nowadays, symbols of maturity such as financial independence from parents and completion of studies are accomplished at later stages. A gradual transition to adult status has some advantages. It gives the young person a longer time in which to develop skills and to prepare for the future, but it tends to produce a period of conflict between dependence and independence. For example, it may be difficult to feel independent living at home supported by your parents.

The development of independence from one's family is a basic task of adolescence. Independence, self-esteem and self-reliance are fostered by parents who lend emotional support and balance the tightrope between authoritarianism and indifference towards their children. In other words, parental responsibility provides support in preparing the youngster for his or her place in the world. Adolescents see themselves as having no more important role in life than to 'find themselves', and will experiment with all kinds of roles in their quest. The identity issues that an adolescent must work out include a career, morality, religion, political ideology and social roles. How an adolescent addresses these issues depends on his level of intellectual thinking at the time.

COGNITIVE DEVELOPMENT

Intellectual development, like everything else in adolescence, occurs at different times in different individuals. This is the final stage of cognitive development, the stage of **formal operations** described by Piaget (see page 9). Not everyone attains this level of mature abstract thought or they may not attain it until early adulthood. Academic achievement depends on whether or not the level of formal operations has been reached; on how the youngster integrates into the school system and on the emphasis the family place on education.

This aspect of development affects the personality. Early maturers tend to be self-confident, calm and are treated maturely by other adolescents and adults. Late maturers tend to be bossy, attention-seeking and restless. However neither early nor late maturity appears to be good or bad in the long run.

Being aware of 'how things are' instead of 'how things might be' may help to explain adolescent moodiness. Conflicts of self-discipline and self-criticism may be resolved by thinking abstractly about the implications of various actions and issues of deep personal concern. Common

Figure 8
Which one is the typical adolescent? *(Reproduced from Chilman and Thomas, 1987)*

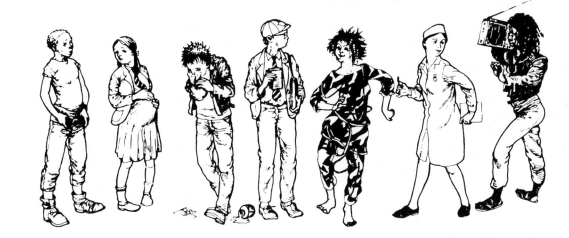

© CHURCHILL LIVINGSTONE 1992 (COPYING BY PERMISSION ONLY)

issues of concern are how we farm animals, environmental issues, religion, wars, love, sex and marriage.

See Exercise 18.

• •

EXERCISE 18

Think about your own adolescence – were there any issues you cared very much about?

(Answers on page 48)

• •

Puberty and the development of secondary sexual characteristics can have an unsettling effect as the adolescent comes to terms with his new identity. Menstruation is a symbol of sexual maturity for a girl so her first experience of this natural physiological event will generally be favourable. Support from a loving mother or carer will reinforce her positive thoughts about it. Similarly, a boy requires loving reassurance and support for his worries over uncontrolled erections and nocturnal ejaculations.

INDEPENDENCE VERSUS DEPENDENCE

Early adolescence, around 11 to 15 years, is when the moods and stresses are worst. The changes occur physically, socially, emotionally and intellectually, but not necessarily in harmony with each other. Young people may resent questions about what they are doing and where they are going. If they feel they are being treated like children there may be family rows, with parents disagreeing with each other or being used one against the other.

The move towards independence may test a parent's patience and understanding but is an essential part of the identity process. The conflict must be resolved without the adolescent feeling isolated, angry or guilty, otherwise they may become alienated. Adolescents may respond to this alienation by finding what they feel is a more meaningful way of life, perhaps by living in a commune or by becoming a single parent. Others may become social dropouts, drug or alcohol abusers, shoplifters or delinquents, or they may develop serious psychological problems such as depression, suicide, hypochondriasis or eating disorders. There are, of course, other reasons for alienation, such as under-achievement or previously unresolved crises of mistrust, shame, guilt and inferiority.

THE MATURE IDENTITY

The gradual appearance of the mature identity occurs after about the 16th birthday. The critical question of 'Who am I'? is resolved with a unique sense of beliefs, values and goals. Moodiness, irritability and self-consciousness are eased with the coming of a new sense of self.

PARENTS VERSUS PEERS

Most adolescents want freedom and most parents want control. Parents may be experiencing their own problems at the same time, perhaps a mid-life crisis, divorce or widowhood. Divorce need not interfere with normal adolescent development if handled well by both partners. Some adolescents may prefer to live with one parent rather than be caught up in constant rows and tears.

How adolescents think about themselves is related to parental attitudes and behaviour. The influence of their own age group grows stronger throughout adolescence. With friends they can test their emerging identity, sexual attractiveness, and generally have a good time with like-minded people. At this time, conflict with friends is usually less than with family members. A compromise is probably the best solution. Those who spend most of their time with friends tend to underachieve at school compared to those who also spend time with family members.

It is probably true that adolescents feel closer to their friends than they do to their parents at this time. However, they may turn to either group for advice if they have a good relationship with both. Within the peer group there may be a 'best friend'. Once young people start dating the opposite sex they tend to rely on their friends for support until after they have been dating for a while, then the 'same sex' friend may become less important.

Having a boy or girlfriend serves several different functions. It is fun and grown up, but it is also an opportunity to consider other people's feelings, accept responsibility and to get along with other people. It can be a morale booster and enhance the individual's self-esteem. In discovering who they find attractive and who finds them attractive, a heterosexual or homosexual identity is formed. A series of temporary relationships gives the young person a chance to explore his sexual identity. The sexual morality of the peer group usually lays down rules for sexual behaviour but most well-adjusted adolescents are also influenced by parental attitudes and values.

Most adolescents become reasonably well-adjusted young adults who look forward to the future with confidence. However, a significant minority take part in various forms of antisocial behaviour.

TEENAGERS – TWO CASE STUDIES

Are adolescents so very troublesome today and is adolescence *really* such a period of storms and stress? A number of studies have found that parents and their teenagers are *not* constantly at odds with each other and it seems that much of the stress which young people show is due to difficulties which their parents are having, for example, marital problems. Also, there isn't a higher incidence of psychiatric disorder amongst this group than any other. Indeed, it seems that depicting adolescents as a problem group is over-emphasising the situation. We are falling into the trap of lumping a group of people together as if they all have the same experiences. Looking at it from the adolescents' point of view, the extent of their 'rebellion' will depend very much on things like their socioeconomic group, their sexuality, their gender and their ethnic origins. The case studies about David and Robert illustrate this point.

We cannot go into these two case studies in any depth; your own response to them will depend on your attitudes and what has shaped them. Maybe you will be able to empathise with this situation,

EXAMPLE

Case Study 1 – David

David is a 16-year-old heterosexual male living in the same town as Robert. However, David lives in the west end of the town in a large detached stone-built villa. He has his own bedroom and attends a public day school in the nearby city. Both his parents work; his father is a doctor in the area.

David has two holidays abroad a year, one skiing during the Christmas holidays, the other in the summer when he usually enjoys practising his windsurfing. He has a good social life sailing in his family's small racing boat and often travels up to the city to be with his school friends and go to a disco at the weekend. David's family and friends expect him to go on to further education of some kind, probably a period of time at university. This will not require any financial sacrifice on anybody's part.

EXAMPLE

Case Study 2 – Robert

Robert is a 16-year-old heterosexual male living in a town on a river renowned for its high rate of unemployment. Certain parts of the town are recognised as areas of high-priority treatment because housing and facilities are regarded as poor. Robert lives in one of the areas of high-priority treatment. His mother does not work and his father cannot find work, although he has tried hard. This is not for the lack of trying.

Robert attends a large local school where his behaviour is very disruptive. His parents are desperately seeking help from every agency they can approach. His father is keen to take him hill-walking and camping but they haven't the money to buy boots, a sleeping bag, waterproof clothing and torch so they can go to the hills in safety.

Neither of Robert's parents enjoyed school and they have difficulty in knowing how to handle the situation now that he is threatened with expulsion. Their expectations of what their children will achieve are different from that of the school and do not necessarily include further education. They are nevertheless horrified that Robert was found taking lead from a local roof, in company with some others, in his leisure time.

The family are receiving state benefit and there is little money for travel, transport or leisure activities. The father is losing his self-esteem; he is very aware that Robert is affected by his inability to find work. This makes him very resentful and he does not appear to hold out much hope for his own future.

that is, 'get inside somebody else's skin and walk about in it for a bit'. **Empathy** does not mean showing pity, or even sympathy, but a deeper understanding which appreciates that any one of us could find ourselves in these situations as a result of birth, poverty, illness or state policies. To feel pity would suggest that the rest of us are in some way 'better' and we are condescending to feel sorry for a moment.

See Exercise 19.

• •

EXERCISE 19

Re-read the case studies but substitute different features. Each time, think how the substitution would affect both the stories and your predictions for each individual's future. For example:

• Make both boys black.
• Make both boys homosexual.
• Substitute girls for boys.

Think about your reactions. Are you aware that you are influenced by what society thinks? How does this affect your relationship with clients?

• •

There is substantial evidence that black people are discriminated against in our society, although we invited black immigrants to our country when we needed their labour in the post-Second World War era. However, a black person with money, privilege and power has a more hopeful future so a black David is more likely to succeed in a material sense than Robert.

If the boys were homosexual the same is probably true. Money provides privilege and power and homosexuality seems to be better tolerated in middle-class society, although it is still regarded as deviant (that is, different from accepted standards).

If we substitute girls for the boys we may find that a female Robert is frowned upon by our society. The socialisation processes at work in our society aim to produce quiet, adaptable females who will not show unusual behaviour but will prepare themselves for their future roles as homemakers and mothers. Studies have shown that girls of all social groups are more likely to be protected and sheltered and less likely to be exposed to danger or criminal activities. (The crime rates for adolescent girls are lower than those for boys.) So, while boys are allowed some licence (and often encouraged to 'sow their wild oats') girls are expected to adopt a much lower profile and rebelliousness is not encouraged.

7

Adulthood

PHYSICAL DEVELOPMENT

It is not easy to identify the changes in physical development that signify adulthood because it is part of the continuous ageing process. Is it reached when adolescence ends, that is, when growth stops because the body has reached its predicted size and shape? Or is it the 'holding' phase when physical skills are practised and maintained before the decline which comes with old age? Adulthood could be both these things – it is certainly a complex subject.

One way of looking at the physical development of the adult is to work out which activities could be called 'adult' activities. First of all, we will identify an adult group.
Try Exercise 20.

When you have finished try to 'sum up' your findings Use this question to help you form a conclusion:

'Is adulthood an extension of adolescence or can I give evidence to support the fact that there is significant physical development associated with adulthood?'

What things have an important influence on the adult's physical well-being? Without the intervention of factors such as disease or injury the hormonal influence, which began at puberty, will programme the development of the adult's physical appearance. As at other stages in life, this development depends on the adult having a healthy lifestyle and a healthy diet.
Try Exercise 21.

EXERCISE 20

Make a note of 10 adults, 5 male and 5 female, in the 20-40 age group. On one side of your paper list their names and ages and make two further columns. Head one 'Occupation' and the other 'Recreational activities'.

The occupation need not be employment-related as some people may not be formally employed, but they will have a daily routine which can be considered an occupation, such as shopping, gardening and housework.

List all the skills each person has developed to carry out the tasks you have identified. Try and work out which of these skills the person developed earlier in life and which he developed later in life. Could the recent skills have been as easily developed at the age of, for example, 15 to 17, in other words, during adolescence?

Try to find someone else who is willing to do the same exercise on their own and then compare notes:

- Discuss what factors would clearly fit into adult physical development.
- What other factors were important in development of the skills?

● ●

EXERCISE 21

List:

- the common injuries which happen to male and female adults

- the common illnesses or conditions that could affect male and female adults

- show your list to colleagues and discuss what short- or long-term effects these incidents might have.

(Answers on page 48)

● ●

All through the development process there are factors which influence normal development. The physical well-being of the adult can be affected by factors such as nutrition, activity and the ability to have adequate rest and sleep.

Other factors, like selection of clothes and footwear, also affect physical well-being. For example, wearing fashionable shoes may cause the early development of problems like bunions or callosities, caused by pressure of ill-fitting footwear. A person's occupation can also influence the development process in adulthood. Both mental and physical development may be affected by stress, the need to be successful, the use of chemicals, gases and other toxic agents as well as the need to adopt habitual postures as in mining, secretarial work and hairdressing.

Intensive physical activity, like that carried out by highly trained athletes or sports enthusiasts, can also produce undesirable physical effects. For example, the surfaces of the joints can show premature signs of excessive wear and tear which limit movement.

Although we can define adulthood as 'the follow-on to adolescence', it is not so easy to decide where the *end* of adulthood occurs. As far as physical development is concerned, adulthood could be defined as 'a life-long process which ends in death, provided the individual is protected from all the factors affecting physical well-being'. However, there are many different opinions about this.

Most parents of young children are in the adult age group. The process of pregnancy and child-bearing is associated with many changes in the body function as the fetus develops from a tiny egg into a baby weighing around 3.5 kilograms (7-8 pounds). This is a normal physiological process but it can cause problems, such as backache, hypertension or high blood pressure and varicose veins; frequency of urinary excretion or constipation are also not uncommon. Many of these problems are temporary. As the fetus grows in size so the abdomen swells and many women retain evidence of their pregnancies in the form of 'stretch marks' because, towards the end of the pregnancy, the skin is excessively stretched.

PSYCHOSOCIAL AND COGNITIVE DEVELOPMENT

Adulthood is the level of development that the individual has been striving for since the beginning of his life. Becoming an adult brings a degree of independence, with rights, privileges and responsibilities not known before. People of either sex can drive a car, drink alcohol, smoke cigarettes, form a sexual relationship, get married, have children, pay income tax and claim social security benefits.

Adults are people who are in charge of their own lives and who accept the responsibility and consequences of their decisions. For some, the transition from adolescence to adulthood can be quick, for others it is a long and gradual process.

THE TRANSITIONAL PERIOD

Maturity does not necessarily occur at the time of emergence from adolescence to adulthood. Maturity signifies the progress of a person's social, emotional and intellectual development in relation to what is expected of people by the society in which we live – almost every day we can learn from new and different experiences.

Certain intellectual abilities reach their climax in early adulthood. Quick response-time, short-term memory and logical abstract thinking, which may not have developed in adolescence, may peak at this stage in life. People who are more intelligent seem to develop this level of formal thought and are capable of processing each new experience to provide new information and valuable insights. The mature adult mind seems to need constant stimulation – each problem encountered and solved is essential to intellectual growth. This has far-reaching consequences for those who enter the adult world without ever having worked.

THE INDEPENDENT ADULT

The self-image of adulthood is increased when independence is achieved – financial and emotional – from one's parents. In doing this, a form of identity crisis develops as we examine who we are and where we are going. We have worked out our adolescent role confusion – we now have to solve the problem of 'intimacy versus isolation'.

Most young people view adulthood as providing opportunities for them to progress in their career, marry, start a family and take their place as a useful member of society. Some young adults may be students, involved in exams and intimate relationships, while others of the same age may be parents, budgeting and bringing up children.

Today's emerging young adult has a wider range of choices to explore alternative lifestyles than previous generations did. The 'eternal adolescent' is in a state of indecision for the best part of his twenties. He strives to find a new identity by indulging in exploratory behaviour. This occurs at all levels of society and may involve drug and alcohol abuse, living rough, travelling, living in a commune or joining a religious group.

Similarly, some adults follow in their parents' footsteps before realising their new self-image is not what they want. Some become committed to political, religious or environmental organisations with totally different viewpoints from those of their parents.

SELF-IMAGE AND IDENTITY

Any change in lifestyle exposes us to conflicting values and emotional choices, such as leaving home or getting married, and this affects our image of ourselves. This is the time when we rely on a strong sense of right or wrong. Our moral development is our personal value system and is related to our intellectual ability and the level of knowledge gained since childhood.

Testing ourselves in the adult world takes place through the contributions we make to others. As we expand into society we make new friends or join groups. We are faced with a variety of situations – friendship, love, hobbies and work. If we fail to gain satisfaction from any of these aspects of our lives our self-esteem and self-image will be affected.

The job we do is of central importance as we take our place in the adult world. Our work provides us with an income – money *we* have *earned*. Self-earned money gives us the freedom to make choices about, for example, how we use our time or what we buy. However, if we are employed we lose a certain amount of freedom and have to adjust to repetition and routine as well as creativity and responsibility. We need to make compromises as we work out our adult lifestyles. It is easy to see why people who are unemployed can lose their self-esteem.

LOVE, MARRIAGE AND PARTNERSHIPS

When two people fall in love they have the opportunity to expand their lives harmoniously together, as well as satisfying their basic sex drives. Many choose a partner, settle down, marry or cohabit in either a heterosexual or homosexual relationship. Others find this neither desirable nor feasible.

People who choose not to commit themselves to a loving relationship do not necessarily run the risk of being isolated. However an intimate relationship with a supportive partner appears to contribute significantly to a person's physical and emotional well-being. People who have someone to share their ideas, feelings and problems with tend to be happier and healthier than those who do not.

More young adults than ever before are cohabiting without legal ties. They do so at a time when they face insecurity and mixed emotions at leaving home and living independently of their parents. This may be the reason why some people also marry at this stage in their lives, although marriage may also be a well-thought-out decision.

Another reason why people marry during these years is their wish to keep in step with their peers. Many of the milestones that mark our progress through life are *expected* to occur at particular times, for example, leaving school, starting work, getting married or having children. These events mark our progress through life but they may occur at different times for different people.

The actual age range for these events varies according to our social class and culture. For instance, Asian girls usually have marriages arranged for them in their late teens. An unemployed person from an unemployed family tends to marry or become a parent earlier than others who may establish their careers first.

See Exercise 22.

EXERCISE 22

- Have you ever been asked by family or friends when are you going to marry or have children?
- How did you feel about the remark?

(Answers on page 48)

Legal marriage vows, made in the presence of witnesses, and perhaps with a religious ceremony, are intended to bind two people for life 'for better or for worse'. This is an important life event showing attachment, conscience and responsibility. Each partner has moved out of his or her own family and created a third.

Living harmoniously develops a mental closeness in a couple whether they are married or not. They find themselves growing into a team, working and solving life's problems together. This may affect their relationship with others. Friendships and family ties may take second place and, sooner or later, sacrifices and compromises have to be made. In this relationship primitive feelings are intimately shared as well as the basic emotions of love and hate. Lovers' quarrels may seem trivial and amusing to the outsider but to the two participants defending their rights they are anything but trivial.

All life events are potentially stressful and require the individual to adapt to a new situation. They may be positive life events, such as marriage, childbirth or job promotion, or negative ones like divorce, bereavement or unemployment. Every individual copes with the same level of stress in different ways – some can be overwhelmed by it, others find it challenging.

As we all experience life events at different ages, the timing and order of our adaptation to adult roles affect the rest of our lives. Similarly, the social support we receive differs from one person to another. By our thirties we have hopefully reached a period of self-assurance and self-sufficiency, knowing what we are capable of doing with our lives and which ambitions we hope to achieve in the future.

SUMMARY EXERCISE

- Choose a popular TV programme which shows life in contemporary Britain.
- Jot down any observations you make from the programme which relate to the issues discussed in this chapter.

(Answers on page 48)

8

The middle years

■ Most of the physical changes which occur during this period, which for convenience we shall take as from approximately 35-60 years, are biological, which means they are related to changes to the body cells and the way they function.

BIOLOGICAL CHANGES

DECLINE IN CELL FUNCTION

In Chapter 1, we discovered that our bodies are made up of millions of cells. Life began with the process of cell division – one cell dividing into two, two into four and so on. This is necessary for the development of a new life and for the growth and maturation of the body. However, during life most of these cells are continually dying and being replaced by identical new cells.

During the periods of fetal growth, infancy, childhood and adolescence the accent is on cell growth. Growth means that few cells are dying, without immediate replacement, and also the cells are functioning to maximum capacity, for example, muscle development as muscles increase in strength. The group of specialised cells which form the brain and nervous system, however, while in abundance and extra to requirements at birth, are not replaced as they wear out and die. This might be quite alarming news to us because we know that the brain is the control centre of the body as a functional unit. From the age of 20 years there is a progressive loss of brain cells.

However, it is reassuring to remember that quality is as important as quantity, so if the cells are developed to their maximum potential the initial loss will be relatively insignificant. Any loss of cells in the brain will have an effect on the body but these changes may not be obvious in early

adulthood. In fact many of the obvious changes are not seen until what we call 'middle age'. While both male and female are affected by the process of cell decline, the changes may be more obvious in one sex than the other at different stages.

MIDDLE AGE

This is the time when the female experiences what is commonly termed 'the change of life' or the **menopause**. Her reproductive period reaches an end because the ovaries start a process of 'run down', almost like a company winding down a business. The process itself may be very gradual or it may be quite sudden. The ovaries produce the female hormones and these hormones bring about body changes, so you can detect the results of their withdrawal. They are seen in the general appearance of the woman, but her health may also be affected as these hormones influence structures like the bones. Lack of hormones can cause reduction in the density of bone over a period of time so that the bones are more readily bent, compressed or broken (osteoporosis).

Because the menopause shows in different ways, individuals are affected differently. Some women have early signs of hormonal withdrawal, for example, their skin becomes wrinkled and loses some of its elastic properties, their breasts tend to sag for the same reason; and their hair may become dry and unmanageable. Many women experience changes in the vagina; it becomes dry of secretions and the resulting irritability can cause intense itching.

Hormonal withdrawal is sometimes given as the reason for unexplained tiredness, irritability, lack of concentration, headaches and sleeplessness. These symptoms are often relieved by **hormone replacement therapy (HRT)**. However, many women do not present any (or many) of these symptoms and often they welcome the menopause because monthly periods (which are often uncomfortable and inconvenient) are no longer a problem.

Males do not appear to go through an obvious 'change of life'. For many men the equivalent 'male menopause', where the ability to reproduce ceases, may not happen until much later in life. Many quite elderly men can father children.

CHANGES IN PHYSICAL APPEARANCE AND ACTIVITY

However, some men may undergo other changes in middle age. It is not uncommon for a man to notice that he is 'thinning on top', the common term for hair loss which can gradually or dramatically lead to balding. This is affected by heredity and tends to run in families. Also, some middle-aged men, like their female counterparts, may feel that they cannot exercise as vigorously as before. For example, instead of two rounds of golf they prefer one; instead of squash they choose a game of badminton. Again, there is no consistent pattern – it is individual to each person. It is true, however, that the high performers, for example, in athletics, tend to be fewer in number at the age of about 50 years. In industry jobs requiring intense activity in, for example, production, have fewer 50 year olds. Perhaps they have progressed up the promotion ladder. Conversely, certain occupations or activities can cause stress-related illness.

PSYCHOSOCIAL AND COGNITIVE DEVELOPMENT

This stage of our lives is often known as the 'prime of life'. Middle age is accompanied by a gradual physical decline from the peak reached in the twenties. The ageing process has been taking place since birth, but now judgment, experience and management ability are valued more than physical strength.

Concerns regarding physical health may become more common in the middle years. Cardiovascular disease and cancer are the two leading causes of death at this time. The emotional and personality factors which lead to stress seem to contribute to health problems in middle age.

COGNITIVE CHANGES

Our knowledge and thought processes should develop further in middle age, if we are influenced by life's experiences, our verbal and social ability, and our moral judgment. Intellectual and manual skills, sharpened by over 20 years of adult living, are keenly sought after. The interaction of intellect and years of information-storing combine to give us wisdom. Our social environment, which affects our attitudes, beliefs and motivation, affects our intellectual functioning too. Those of us who are socially active tend to increase our intellectual ability, or **generate**, but if we are socially isolated there is a tendency to decline or **stagnate**.

PSYCHOSOCIAL DEVELOPMENT

This is a time of considerable adjustment in areas of self, family relations, social interactions, career development and leisure time. It is often referred to as 'the mid-life crisis'. Most of us find ourselves the middle generation with responsibilities to elderly parents and older children. After years of sharing our lives with children we may find ourselves alone, having resolved the adolescent conflicts with them. The 'empty nest' phase of the family life cycle signifies freedom. However, for some the absence of the children is hard to bear.

Many wives and mothers experience some degree of restlessness or dissatisfaction with their home-making role. With more free time, many re-enter employment, increase their work hours, enrol for courses, or take up voluntary work or a leisure activity. Middle-aged women are likely to be more committed to their employment as their marriage or family goal has been achieved.

In many respects, life changes for the better with many couples enjoying being childless again. Time for travel, holidays, having a night out without babysitters or a chance to be alone together can strengthen a waning relationship. Some couples drift apart now as other opportunities come their way. Divorce is a common cause of mid-life stress.

For single people and for married couples it is a time for reflection, thinking about what could have been and what has been achieved. They want the best for the next generation and some people may assume social or civic responsibility to achieve this aim. Becoming a grandparent plays an important role in lending intellectual, social and emotional support to the extended family. As we are likely to be at the peak of our earning power this is a time when the extended family can be indulged a little.

Marital adjustment is essential after the children leave home. Successful marriages take many forms, from couples who are totally involved with each other to others whose bickering and fighting keep them going! Marital relations are often under stress during the middle years. Sexual satisfaction may decrease while pressures from work, redundancy or career changes may increase. Similar interests, attitudes, and companionship involving mutual caring, trust and open communication are all important to a continuing marriage. People with personality traits which include emotional maturity, self-esteem, adaptability, consideration for others and the ability to express affection tend to succeed at marriage.

Divorce at any age is a painful, stressful event for all concerned and is usually followed by some loss of self-esteem, loneliness and alterations in lifestyle. Most divorced people do remarry and most of these remarriages are successful. Those who remarry are likely to have lowered their expectations or altered their attitudes, and tend to value companionship and affection before anything else.

Think about this further in Exercise 23.

EXERCISE 23

If you know any clients, relatives or friends who are remarried and who would be willing to talk about their experiences, ask them about their priorities in their remarriage.

Widowhood is often a middle-aged event. If experienced at this time of life it may be combined with children leaving home or with bringing up adolescents as a single parent. This leads to a combination of stressful life events and the effect on the individual can be quite devastating.

SUMMARY EXERCISE

The number of 'Well man' and 'Well woman' clinics has greatly increased recently. Why is this particularly appropriate to middle-aged men and women who currently live in Britain?

To answer this question you can use the information in this chapter, research what is publicised in the media, or find out what services local health authority workers have to offer this age group.

(Answers on page 48)

9

The older adult

The idea of 'old age' causes much argument and discussion. Many people think it means the same as retirement. As with adolescence and adulthood, it is difficult to define where adulthood ends and old age starts. Perhaps it is impossible to draw such a line clearly. There are many factors which make it difficult to define what is meant by old age, including the influence of heredity, environment, geographic location and culture. Perhaps it is more useful to examine what changes are likely to become obvious from the time of formal retirement.

THEORIES OF AGEING

Many theories are used to explain the physical changes which start around the period of middle years and progress until death. One is the biological theory of the **life cycle**. This theory says that from birth there is a period of growth and development which peaks in early adulthood and is followed by a levelling off, or a plateau, where no significant change takes place; this is followed by a gradual process of decline, or degeneration, until death.

Another theory suggests that the repetitive process of cell division has an influence on the ageing process. When cells divide by the process of reduplication the 'photocopy' becomes less accurate in advancing years. This is termed **cell mutation**. If these cells become less specialised, it follows that the tissues and organs made up of these groups of cells will deteriorate in functional ability. Consequently, this process of decline produces changes which can be observed.

Think about this in relation to a machine, such as a motor car. As the car ages, the battery becomes less efficient and the engine is more difficult to start; the tyres get worn so that the car does not function well on the road; the bodywork loses its protective coating and may show signs of rust; the engine parts wear and the engine burns oil which can be seen in the exhaust gas. We do know, however, that if the car is carefully tended by the owner then this process can be slowed down considerably. Also, a car specialist can replace worn out parts, as they suffer wear and tear or damage, with new parts so that the whole car continues to function well. This is now possible, if only to a limited extent, in the human body. Perhaps you can think about some examples yourself. Later in the chapter we shall investigate to what extent the ageing process can be delayed in the human being.

Before we explore further the changes associated with ageing, take a look at what it consists of and how it is seen by different people.

See Exercise 24.

● ●

EXERCISE 24

- Look at your physical state, the appearance of your body and how it functions for you now. Make a list of the features you think you might have when you are 65 and 75 years old. Share these predictions with members of your group. What are your conclusions?
- Try and find a person you can interview from each of the following age groups:

  10-16; 16-19; 20-25; 26-30; 30-40; 41-50; 51-60; 61-70; 71-75; 76-80; 81-90.

  Ask each of them the following questions (and others of your own choice). You could tape-record their responses, if they are willing.
  - When do they think someone is 'old'?
  - What sort of activities are they involved in during a typical day?
  - Is there anything they would like to tell you about their life?
  - What do they enjoy doing in their leisure time?
  - Is there anything they would like to be able to do which they cannot do without assistance?

- Can your friends guess the age of each interviewee from his or her response?

● ●

Exercise 24 will help you to appreciate the physical changes associated with ageing so you can identify its positive aspects as well as the problem areas.

THE BIOLOGICAL PROCESS OF AGEING

SKIN

As the skin loses its elasticity it becomes lined and wrinkled. This is particularly noticeable in the face, neck, arms and hands although the whole body is gradually affected. The skin appears to be thinner and sometimes underlying structures such as blood vessels become more prominent.

MUSCLES

Muscles which were highly developed in adolescence and adulthood gradually lose their tone, unless the individual exercises continuously to maintain their function. As a result, they are less able to support the skeleton in the upright position and this causes the body to stoop. Also, the front part of the abdominal cavity is made up largely of muscle so that deterioration in the muscle function here produces the characteristic 'paunch' or 'corporation' which is more obvious in men, although they may attempt to conceal it! This loss of muscle bulk and tone also affects the general appearance, particularly in areas like the upper arms and thighs where these muscles were once well developed; the skin sags and appears 'baggy'; in the face, loss of muscle tone gives the face a 'fallen' appearance and there may be 'bags' around the eyes.

Internal muscles also lose their tone. The female, in the post-menopausal period in particular, may experience specific symptoms. The uterus, once well supported by muscles, begins to sag and may press on the bladder and bowel giving rise to symptoms of stress incontinence (occasional uncontrolled dribbling of urine). As the pelvic floor muscles also sag these conditions increase.

Even the muscles which control the voice box during speech are affected and sometimes you can hear a voice change as people get older; the voice may become hoarse, thickened or roughened; conversely, it may become more high-pitched depending on whether the vocal cords are being relaxed or stretched by the effects of muscle and cartilage worsening in quality (known as **degeneration**).

SKELETON

The bony skeleton, the framework of the body, loses some of its structural content. This means that bones are more easily broken. Between the bones of the spine the discs, made of softer cartilage, which cushion the spine against jarring and injury, are also likely to worsen in quality. This means that as well as the spinal bones (vertebrae) themselves collapsing, the less functional discs reduce in size; so the body height appears to shorten and the tendency to stoop is exaggerated.

EYES

The cells which allow the eyes to focus on objects, for example, in reading, writing or knitting, function less well and reading glasses may have to be used. While many young people need to wear glasses to correct visual defects, the defects are not quite the same as the problem of ageing eyes which is called **presbyopia.**

EARS

A similar lowering in quality takes place in the ears, where the highly specialised cells which pick up the sensations of sound become more sluggish. This leads to varying degrees of hearing difficulty, the worst being deafness. It is important to remember that there are other causes of deafness, like solidified wax in the ears, and these should be investigated and treated.

JOINTS

The freely movable joints, where two or more bones meet, are covered by a smooth layer of cartilage and supported by a joint capsule containing the joint fluid. These are the joints that are used in highly active daily routines, whether at work or play. It is not surprising, therefore, that the years of wear and tear take their toll sooner or later, giving rise to the condition known as **osteoarthritis**, which causes pain and joint stiffness. Stiffness of the joints is particularly troublesome in the weight-bearing joints of the hips, knees and ankles.

Other joints, like those of the spine, involved in daily tasks of lifting, carrying, pushing and pulling, are also affected by wear and tear, and stiffness is again a problem. The result is slowness of movement referred to as a 'reduction in mobility'. Other problems follow from the lack of mobility. Loss of bone density, called **osteoporosis**, makes the bones more brittle as the bone structure gets thinner. This means that bones are weaker than before and so more easily fractured or broken.

CIRCULATION

The effective circulation of blood around the body depends primarily on good heart function. It is also assisted by the action of the body muscles which act like a pump to encourage the circulation as these muscles contract and relax during everyday activity. A reduction in activity, therefore, will make the circulatory process more sluggish. If, at the same time, there are degenerative changes in the heart the situation is made worse. The signs are paleness of the skin, intolerance of cold temperatures, tiredness and sometimes

breathlessness. Normally, the muscles of the skin contract vigorously in cold temperatures and we shiver. If these muscles do not function effectively the older person cannot shiver in order to generate heat.

Poor circulation also affects other areas of the body which depend on the circulation for food and oxygen. For example, the brain may be less functional not only because of degeneration in the nerve cells but also because of poorer circulation.

TEETH AND HAIR

Other features not uncommon as the ageing process advances include the loosening and loss of teeth, not necessarily because of decay but due to the gums receding and the fixation of the teeth in the jaws becoming less secure. The distribution of hair over the body may appear more sparse as, for example, pubic and axillary hair gets thinner. However, some females develop hair, particularly in the male beard area. This is due to the effects of hormone withdrawal: the natural female hormones no longer balance the smaller levels of male hormone in the body.

DELAYING THE AGEING PROCESS

So that you do not get a totally depressing picture about the older adult it is a good idea to find out why many people in this age group seem to conserve their youth and do not look their age. Many people set out on new ventures and open up new horizons when they retire; they don't really retire at all but change occupations. What factors influence the delay or acceleration of the ageing process?
See Exercise 25.

● ●

EXERCISE 25

List things you have come across in relation to people you know or have worked with which can make them age:

– more gradually
– more quickly.

You could list your answers in 3 columns:

● Health   ● Lifestyle   ● Diet

(Answers on page 48)

● ●

THE STATUS OF ELDERLY PEOPLE

Too often, elderly people with wrinkles, grey hair, baldness, a stoop, delicate loose skin and a limp due to an osteoarthritic hip are viewed quite negatively by the younger generation, almost as if their appearance is unacceptable. Perhaps it is important for younger people to be aware of what these signs of age stand for. Could they be considered worthwhile marks of experience, showing a person who has solved many of life's problems, gained wisdom and who is now a historian with first-hand knowledge of past times? This would certainly generate positive thinking so that the elderly person would cherish their physical status rather than try to hide or camouflage it, something which is both time-consuming and expensive.

PSYCHOSOCIAL AND COGNITIVE DEVELOPMENT

As more of our population live longer, and the number of aged people increases, our need for understanding this final stage of human development becomes greater.

RETIREMENT

Activities

The retirement age from paid employment is still officially 65 years for men and 60 years for women. Many people take early retirement; others, especially those in positions of authority such as family businessmen or judges, may work on. For many people retirement is marked by withdrawal from money-earning work. Some people may not have worked for years, having been chronically unemployed, made redundant or too ill to work. Our self-identity revolves around who we are and what we do – a doctor, a policeman, a businessman, a labourer, a care worker, a teacher or unemployed. With retirement this identity is taken from us, generally along with a good deal of our income too.

There is, however, a positive side to retirement if it is seen as a time to develop new skills and leisure activities. Many in this age group have the health to enjoy holidays at home or abroad, or take up long-standing or new interests which previously they had little time to pursue. Some seize the opportunity for further intellectual achievement, like studying for academic awards such as diplomas or degrees. All these activities help to keep the person 'young'.

Relationships

The retirement period is generally associated with high marital satisfaction for both partners. The adjustment to companionship found in the middle years seems complete. Married people experience less loneliness and the quality of their life together is usually good. Sexual performance is not as important as sharing sexual pleasure. 'Sharing' would appear to be the keyword to success and domestic chores are often shared as part of the daily routine.

Most elderly people live independently but near to their children. They may rely on them in times of illness and stress. This can be a two-way process, with advice and emotional support being given as well as received.

Relationships with grandchildren vary considerably and usually depend on the quality of family relationships built up over the years. Grandparents are not burdened with the responsibility of parents and the generation gap can be bridged successfully, giving a great deal of pleasure and wisdom to both parties. The grandparent may have held the family together during a divorce or single parent upbringing. Older people who have never married or had a family seem to adapt to old age alone just as they adapted to being alone in previous years. They may have had to come to terms with the death of their own elderly parents or siblings (brothers and sisters) but they are spared the trauma of widowhood.

Widowhood represents the greatest of all emotional and social losses suffered by individuals. It may have occurred in early or middle adulthood but the majority are widowed at 60 and over. Like divorce, it is an experience which has to be lived through although the altered social status can be hard to accept.

BEREAVEMENT

Bereavement should follow a natural process. Physical symptoms of loss of appetite and sleep are followed by numbed shock, anger, quiet disbelief and despair. Contemplation of the individual's own death may be accompanied by a variety of health problems and anxieties until finally a stage of acceptance and adjustment is reached. The whole process may take a year or two and there is an increased incidence of mortality in spouses during this period.

The stages of adjustment may involve living alone, remarrying, living with relatives or entering residential care. The course chosen depends very much on the person's state of mental and physical health and his or her ability to make the adjustment. Part of the achievement of independence is staying in the same home, at least for a time, surrounded by memories during this crucial stage of readjustment.

Most elderly people seem to prefer to live alone despite the problems of loneliness and isolation. Many may need considerable community resources to allow them to achieve this aim. Generally, those who enter residential care do so when their physical and mental frailty dictates and because other care is unavailable. Bereavement often triggers off the process of disengagement.

DISENGAGEMENT

We often say we would like to grow old gracefully, meaning to slow down or 'fail' naturally – this is called **disengagement**. Activities of daily living and socialisation become less and a person's circle of friends becomes smaller. There is a mutual withdrawal, in that society also expects less of the elderly person. Accompanied by this social withdrawal is a preoccupation with self and decreased interest in those around us and in the environment. The physical ageing process will, to a certain extent, dictate the age at which an elderly person disengages, and wide variations exist according to our state of health. Heart disease, bone disease, memory loss, sensory loss and bereavement may all speed up this process. Our personalities, moulded throughout life, contribute to the way in which we cope with disengagement.

COGNITIVE CHANGES

As bodily functions continue to decline, incapacity and illness can be deeply depressing. Deterioration of brain function causes intellectual and sensory impairment as well as affecting physical processes such as walking or balance. Communication may be a problem, caused by deafness or loss of speech, for example, with stroke victims. Eyesight may be so poor that the person can no longer read, adding to his frustration. Thought processes may become confused by the severe frustration of impairment and helpers can be made to feel hurt or embarrassed in their attempts to help.

Recently, it has been suggested that Piaget's stages of cognitive development are repeated in old age, in reverse order! Have you ever compared an elderly person to a self-centred child? Elderly people who live alone, or who may not have a friend of relative nearby with whom to discuss their thoughts and fears, will tend to become more self-centred. Disengagement is also closely linked with intellectual deterioration.

Compared to young adults, old people perform poorly on problem-solving and may respond to previously learned issues as if they were new. Memory loss accounts for some of this impairment. Recent events are frequently forgotten whereas childhood memories may be very vivid. On the other hand, many old people function very well in the everyday world and may 'tick by' for many years. Some may hold down jobs beyond the official retirement age. These tend to be people who realise their creativity and wisdom is a much sought after commodity.

See Exercise 26.

● ●

EXERCISE 26

- Think about people you know or have read about who fall into the following categories:

• dentists	• home helps	• cabinet ministers
• electricians	• judges	• family businessmen
• insurance agents	• factory workers	• university lecturers

You could add some other professions and occupations yourself.

- Compare the retirement age of each occupation.
- Are some compelled to retire at 60 or 65?
- Which of them had the opportunity to continue to work and had the choice of when to retire from work?
- How would you account for the differences between them?

● ●

Some older adults have a brain disorder or a progressive disease which influences their intellectual abilities. Most disorders produce similar symptoms although the severity of the symptoms varies from slight to profound, and their progression from slow to rapid.

Many problems, like learning difficulties, judgmental problems, disorientation and emotional lability (unpredictable control of emotions, for example, crying) are found at other transition stages, like adolescence. However, they recur more frequently with age with the added symptom of memory loss. These symptoms indicate that the brain, or mental processing, is less effective than it had been earlier in life; this is termed **cerebral dysfunction** and it may be acute or chronic.

In acute dysfunction, physical diseases may be the cause, for example, infection, 'hardening' of the arteries or **arteriosclerosis**, an alteration in the body chemistry or electrolyte imbalance, alcoholism or drug toxicity. These threatening situations can produce persecutory feelings and personality changes, as the natural social skills of a lifetime's experience fall away. Dependence on others may be bitterly resisted.

DEATH

We do not know what death is, or what developmental significance it has for us. In recent years, mainly thanks to hospice terminal care, dying has become an acknowledged and accepted part of life and no longer a taboo subject.

One theory now being considered is that dying is not usually a distinct moment in time, when a person changes from alive to dead (although sudden death may be like this). Even in the absence of incurable disease, dying is part of a process in elderly people. They anticipate dying and this is reinforced by the death of spouses and peers.

Generally there is a final deterioration of physical and intellectual skills when the elderly person is described as 'failing'. Five stages of adjustment to the dying process have been described by a researcher named Elizabeth Kubler-Ross. These are shown in the panel in the right-hand column.

Not everyone progresses through these psychological stages and death may intervene at any time. These attitudes probably reflect the attitudes of those of any age who have come to terms with having a terminal illness. An elderly person may only experience depression and acceptance before death. If he can reflect on a useful, worthwhile life he may not want to live longer, especially if his spouse and many of his peers have died. Many old people take pride in having their affairs in order or having enough money for their funeral. With death, the cycle of life is complete.

THE DYING PROCESS – KUBLER-ROSS

- **Stage 1** – Denial and isolation
  Reaction is 'It cannot be me'

- **Stage 2** – Anger
  Reaction is 'Why me?'

- **Stage 3** – Bargaining
  Reaction is to change one's attitude in return for 'more time'

- **Stage 4** – Depression
  As the body fails and becomes weaker the sense of loss of life is felt and the person expresses their feelings and sorrow.

- **Stage 5** – Acceptance
  Death is accepted as inevitable and the person is often peaceful and calm. He sleeps often and is tired. Frequently the person detaches himself from reality and death is not talked about.

- -

SUMMARY EXERCISE

Find some family photographs which show more than one generation. If you can, try to find pictures of people in the following age groups:

- newborn
- infancy
- childhood
- adolescent
- adult
- middle age
- retirement

- Can you pinpoint the characteristic features of each stage in life?
- Why are there differences or similarities between people of the same age group?
- What do the pictures tell you about each era?

Suggested things to look for:

– do they look healthy?
– what is significant about their dress?
– who are they with or what are they doing in the pictures?

(Answers on page 48)

- -

REFERENCES

Kubler-Ross E 1969 On death and dying.
McMillan, New York

SUGGESTED READING

Atkinson D, Williams F (Eds) 1990 Know me as
I am (an anthology of prose, poetry and art by
people with learning difficulties). Hodder and
Stoughton, London (in association with the
Open University)

Barnes A 1991 Personal and community health 3E.
Ballière Tindall, London

Bond J, Bond S 1986 Sociology and health care.
Churchill Livingstone, Edinburgh

Browne K, Davies C & Stratton P 1988 Early
prediction and prevention of child abuse.
Wiley and Sons, Lancaster

Dickson A 1992 Menopause, the woman's view –
a change for the better. Quartet, London

Prince J, Adams M 1987 The Psychology of
childbirth 2E. Churchill Livingstone, Edinburgh

Roberts M, Tamurrini J 1981 Child development
0-5. Holmes McDougall, Edinburgh

Shaw M 1991 The challenge of ageing 2E.
Churchill Livingstone, Edinburgh

Sheridan M 1983 From birth to five years –
children's developmental progress. Nelson,
London

Smith R 1987 Unemployment and health – a
disaster and a challenge. Oxford University
Press, Oxford

Wilson K 1990 Ross & Wilson Anatomy and
physiology in health and illness 7E. Churchill
Livingstone, Edinburgh

ANSWERS

Ch. 1 – Summary Ex C, C, A, B, A, A, D, B

Ch. 2 - Ex 4

Experts could include:

JANET – teacher, school nurse, doctor, child/educational psychologist, optician, specialist teacher

JOHN – teacher, school nurse, doctor, child/educational psychologist, speech therapist, specialist medical paediatrician (plus possibility of referral to hospital)

Ch. 3 – Ex 6 – It is the *male* who determines the sex of the fetus because only he can contribute the Y chromosome representing maleness.

Ex 7 – The sperm enter the vaginal canal, are propelled up through the cavity of the uterus into the uterine, or fallopian, tube and there meet with the ovum. Fertilisation takes place here. The main site of growth and development is the uterus (or womb).

If fertilisation does not occur the egg is discharged from the uterus in the next menstrual flow (period).

Fertilisation is more likely to be successful about 12-16 days from the last menstrual period. Some of the causes of infertility are: faulty development of ova or sperm, blockages in the fallopian/uterine tubes, obesity, ill-health, low sperm count, failure to ovulate

– Ex 8

- **DISORDER : SICKLE-CELL ANAEMIA**
  - CAUSE : **Genetic – recessive gene**
  - EFFECT : **Failure to thrive, jaundice, recurrent infections**
  - ACTION : **If acute crisis occurs, hospitalisation for oxygen, IV therapy and pain relief**

- **DISORDER : DOWN'S SYNDROME**
  - CAUSE : **Chromosomal abnormality**
  - EFFECT : **Do not have the same development potential as an unaffected child – slower mental, physical and intellectual development**
  - ACTION : **Extra intellectual and social stimulation**

- **DISORDER : HAEMOPHILIA**
  - CAUSE : **Genetic – X-linked, from female carrier to male sufferer**
  - EFFECT : **Excessive bleeding from 'minor' injuries – restricts play, frequent hospital visits**
  - ACTION : **Administration of factor VIII which is missing from the blood**

- **DISORDER : SPINA BIFIDA**
  - CAUSE : **Unknown**
  - EFFECT : **Neural tube defect in fetal life. If severe, child may spend his life in a wheelchair**
  - ACTION : **Initial surgery may be needed.**

All individuals affected by these disorders also benefit from specialist support from the community – midwife, health visitor, psychologist, social worker, GP, voluntary agencies and support groups.

– **Ex 9 – Weeks 1-14** - frequent passing or urine, morning sickness, fullness of breasts, increase in size of uterus
Weeks 15-28 – fetal movements, abdominal enlargement, pressure i.e. feelings of cramp
Weeks 29-40 – very obviously pregnant, perhaps sudden alteration in shape when baby drops further into the pelvis, intermittent mild uterine contractions

– **Ex 10 – • Labour** – when developed fetus is delivered from the protection of the mother's uterus to sustain its own independent life in the outside world

• **Start of labour:**
– release of 'plug' of blood-stained mucous followed by regular rhythmic contractions (or contractions followed by blood-stained discharge)
– the bag of fluid surrounding the baby ruptures ('breaking of the waters') followed by regular contractions
• **Time** – varies. First pregnancies (primigravida) may take several hours; subsequent pregnancies take less time because muscles have been previously stretched
3 stages:
– dilation of the cervix, so baby's head can emerge
– expulsion, where mother physically assists the automatic action of her uterine muscles to 'push' the baby through the birth canal
– expulsion of the placenta (afterbirth)

– **Ex 13** – Lack of: HEARING – delayed speech; SIGHT – delayed recognition of objects and their function; slow to smile; TASTE – inhibits the enjoyment of food; chewing might be less intuitive; might delay weaning; SMELL – delays child's appreciation of signals in the environment e.g. food cooking, smell of burning; could prove to be hazardous; TOUCH – delays sensory motor development e.g. inability to recognise temperature, texture, physical contact injuries may occur of which child is unaware

Ch. 4 – Ex 12

DEVELOPMENT CHART

MONTHS	POSTURE AND LARGE MOTOR SKILLS	HEARING AND LANGUAGE	VISION AND FINE MOTOR SKILLS	SOCIAL BEHAVIOUR AND PLAY
0				
1				Sucks thumb
2		Social smiles		
3	Lifts head above	Coos or	Discovers fingers	Eats from spoon
4	shoulders	gurgles	Follows objects moving before eyes	
5	Rolls from back to front			Turns eyes to sound
6	Sits up with	Chuckles when played with	Palmar grasp	
7	support	Vocalises 'Da Da'	Holds on to rattle	
8		'Ma Ma'	Holds object in both hands	First teeth appear
9				Shy of strangers
10	Crawls or moves from spot		Uses index finger	
11	Holds on to furniture		Pincer group	
12				
13	Takes first steps			
14				
15				
16				Drinks from a cup
17				
18				
Years				
2				
3				
4				
5				

Ch. 6 – Ex 18 – not given the opportunity to enter into adult conversation or contribution ignored

– when going out – having to account for whereabouts and exact time will be home

– not having charge over own finances

– told what to do in the home, rather than being consulted adult to adult

– **Ex 21 – Injuries** – burns, fractures (broken leg, crushed fingers, spinal or head injuries), damaged muscles or tendons

Illness – high blood pressure; heart attack; chronic bronchitis; anaemia; obesity; disorders of an organ or system of the body like asbestosis; AIDS; hepatitis These may have traumatic effects on lifestyle e.g. a change of occupation or house; constant medical attention

– **Ex 22** – • Annoyed, embarrassed, insulted, amused

• Censored for not conforming to the 'norm'

• Credited for having an individual view

– **Summary Ex** – Soap operas like 'Neighbours' or 'Coronation Street' include: forming a lasting relationship v. isolation; stressful family events; starting a family; intellectual peak

Ch. 8 – Summary Ex – Greater awareness of effect of lifestyle on health

– White Paper emphasis on prevention of ill-health/health concerns

– Advice from health workers

Ch. 9 – Ex 25 – Gradually:

• **Health** – free from disease and injury; access to adequate fresh air and sunshine; ability to cope with the problems of daily living without being overstressed

• **Lifestyle** – comfortable, dry, warm accommodation; enough money for food and clothing; access to personal cleanliness

• **Diet** – necessary nutrition for body building/maintenance and for avoidance of under/over eating.

Quickly: Those who do not enjoy good health, mental or physical, tend to age more quickly

– **Summary Ex** –

• Characteristics – physique, muscular development, body shape, posture, teeth, hair

• Differences/similarities – genetic or due to environmental influences

• Changes – attitudes to dress from formal to informal, economic status, striking social class differences, occupations and implications about gender roles, extended family more in evidence

NOTES

NOTES